CA

D1559972

Food Allergies and Sensitivities

Recent Titles in
Q&A Health Guides

Self-Injury: Your Questions Answered
Romeo Vitelli

Living Green: Your Questions Answered
Amy Hackney Blackwell

Sexually Transmitted Diseases: Your Questions Answered
Paul Quinn

Mindfulness and Meditation: Your Questions Answered
Blaise Aguirre

Anxiety and Panic Disorders: Your Questions Answered
Daniel Zwillenberg

Substance Abuse: Your Questions Answered
Romeo Vitelli

Eating Disorders: Your Questions Answered
Justine J. Reel

Food Allergies and Sensitivities

Your Questions Answered

Alice C. Richer

Q&A Health Guides

GREENWOOD™

An Imprint of ABC-CLIO, LLC
Santa Barbara, California • Denver, Colorado

Copyright © 2019 by ABC-CLIO, LLC

All rights reserved. No part of this publication may be reproduced, stored in a retrieval system, or transmitted, in any form or by any means, electronic, mechanical, photocopying, recording, or otherwise, except for the inclusion of brief quotations in a review, without prior permission in writing from the publisher.

Library of Congress Cataloging-in-Publication Data

Names: Richer, Alice C., author.
Title: Food allergies and sensitivities : your questions answered / Alice C. Richer.
Description: Santa Barbara, California : ABC-CLIO, LLC/Greenwood, [2019] | Series: Q&A health guides | Includes bibliographical references and index.
Identifiers: LCCN 2018040017 (print) | LCCN 2018041380 (ebook) | ISBN 9781440856358 (ebook) | ISBN 9781440856341 (print : alk. paper)
Subjects: | MESH: Food Hypersensitivity | Food Intolerance
Classification: LCC RC596 (ebook) | LCC RC596 (print) | NLM WD 310 | DDC 616.97/5—dc23
LC record available at https://lccn.loc.gov/2018040017

ISBN: 978-1-4408-5634-1 (print)
978-1-4408-5635-8 (ebook)

23 22 21 20 19 1 2 3 4 5

This book is also available as an eBook.

Greenwood
An Imprint of ABC-CLIO, LLC

ABC-CLIO, LLC
147 Castilian Drive
Santa Barbara, CA 93117
www.abc-clio.com

This book is printed on acid-free paper ∞

Manufactured in the United States of America

For Pete, Mike, and Dan, whose support is immeasurable.
For Carrie and Lauren, who struggle with food allergies.

Contents

Series Foreword

All of us have questions about our health. Is this normal? Should I be doing something differently? Whom should I talk to about my concerns?

And our modern world is full of answers. Thanks to the Internet, there's a wealth of information at our fingertips, from forums where people can share their personal experiences to Wikipedia articles to the full text of medical studies. But finding the right information can be an intimidating and difficult task—some sources are written at too high a level, others have been oversimplified, while still others are heavily biased or simply inaccurate.

Q&A Health Guides address the needs of readers who want accurate, concise answers to their health questions, authored by reputable and objective experts, and written in clear and easy-to-understand language.

This series focuses on the topics that matter most to young adult readers, including various aspects of physical and emotional well-being as well as other components of a healthy lifestyle. These guides will also serve as a valuable tool for parents, school counselors, and others who may need to answer teens' health questions.

All books in the series follow the same format to make finding information quick and easy. Each volume begins with an essay on health literacy and why it is so important when it comes to gathering and evaluating health information. Next, the top five myths and misconceptions that surround the topic are dispelled. The heart of each guide is a collection of questions and answers, organized thematically. A selection of five case studies provides real-world examples to illuminate key concepts. Rounding out each volume are a directory of resources, glossary, and index.

It is our hope that the books in this series will not only provide valuable information but will also help guide readers toward a lifetime of healthy decision making.

Introduction

The number of people who struggle with food allergies, intolerances, and sensitivities has increased over the past few decades. The World Allergy Organization estimates that as of 2013 approximately 220–250 million people worldwide struggled with at least one food allergy. The Food Allergy Research and Education organization reports childhood food allergies increased approximately 50 percent from 1977 through 2011 in the United States. Health-care providers worldwide also report increased cases of adverse food reactions.

Symptoms range from mild to chronically debilitating to life threatening, and the impact of them is significant, both personally and financially. The Americans with Disabilities Act of 1990 now includes those who live with adverse food reactions, and medical costs for the treatment of children in the United States with food allergies are an estimated $25 billion annually.

Although most people assume all food reactions are allergies, this is not the case. True food allergies involve the immune system and is frequently life threatening. An estimated 90 percent of food allergies worldwide are to eggs, cow's milk, legumes (peanuts, beans), sesame seeds, shellfish, soy, tree nuts, and wheat. However, any food can cause an allergy in susceptible individuals. Food intolerances and sensitivities are distinguished from food allergies because they rarely involve the immune system, are often chronic and debilitating, and are thought to be the root cause for many chronic illnesses. It is yet to be determined exactly why an individual becomes allergic, intolerant, or sensitive to a food, but there are many different theories.

Current testing methods used to diagnose a food allergy or intolerance reaction have an estimated 50–60 percent accuracy rate. However, testing methods for food sensitivities remain unreliable at best. Treatment options vary and are based on individual symptoms. Public health concerns are many regarding the safety of an allergic individual. One strategy to protect allergic individuals is to ban peanuts and tree nuts from public places. This has resulted in unintended consequences while also impacting those who do not have food allergies. Food safety laws have also been enacted to protect allergic individuals. Research on adverse food reactions has steadily increased since the 1970s and is ongoing in the areas of more accurate testing methods and new treatment methods.

The objective of this book is to provide information and education that help to easily distinguish between food allergies, food intolerances, and food sensitivities. It also answers the questions many people have about adverse food reactions, how to manage them, and reviews the most recent, accurate, scientific evidence available in an easy-to-understand format. How the medical community came to understand adverse food reactions is explored. Symptoms, treatment, and testing methods are discussed as well as the impact food allergies, intolerances, and sensitivities have on individuals and families. Support group information is provided along with a listing of resources for further information.

Guide to Health Literacy

On her 13th birthday, Samantha was diagnosed with type 2 diabetes. She consulted her mom and her aunt, both of whom also have type 2 diabetes, and decided to go with their strategy of managing diabetes by taking insulin. As a result of participating in an after-school program at her middle school that focused on health literacy, she learned that she can help manage the level of glucose in her bloodstream by counting her carbohydrate intake, following a diabetic diet, and exercising regularly. But what exactly should she do? How does she keep track of her carbohydrate intake? What is a diabetic diet? How long should she exercise and what type of exercise should she do? Samantha is a visual learner, so she turned to her favorite source of media, YouTube, to answer these questions. She found videos from individuals around the world sharing their experiences and tips, doctors (or at least people who have "Dr." in their YouTube channel names), government agencies such as the National Institutes of Health, and even video clips from cat lovers who have cats with diabetes. With guidance from the librarian and the health and science teachers at her school, she assessed the credibility of the information in these videos and even compared their suggestions to some of the print resources that she was able to find at her school library. Now, she knows exactly how to count her carbohydrate level, how to prepare and follow a diabetic diet, and how much (and what) exercise is needed daily. She intends to share her findings with her mom and her aunt, and now she wants to create a chart that summarizes what she has learned that she can share with her doctor.

Samantha's experience is not unique. She represents a shift in our society; an individual no longer views himself or herself as a passive recipient of medical care but as an active mediator of his or her own health. However, in this era when any individual can post his or her opinions and experiences with a particular health condition online with just a few clicks or publish a memoir, it is vital that people know how to assess the credibility of health information. Gone are the days when "publishing" health information required intense vetting. The health information landscape is highly saturated, and people have innumerable sources where they can find information about practically any health topic. The sources (whether print, online, or a person) that an individual consults for health information are crucial because the accuracy and trustworthiness of the information can potentially affect his or her overall health. The ability to find, select, assess, and use health information constitutes a type of literacy—health literacy—that everyone must possess.

THE DEFINITION AND PHASES OF HEALTH LITERACY

One of the most popular definitions for health literacy comes from Ratzan and Parker (2000), who describe health literacy as "the degree to which individuals have the capacity to obtain, process, and understand basic health information and services needed to make appropriate health decisions." Recent research has extrapolated health literacy into health literacy bits, further shedding light on the multiple phases and literacy practices that are embedded within the multifaceted concept of health literacy. Although this research has focused primarily on online health information seeking, these health literacy bits are needed to successfully navigate both print and online sources. There are six phases of health information seeking: (1) information need identification and question formulation, (2) information search, (3) information comprehension, (4) information assessment, (5) information management, and (6) information use.

The first phase is the *information need identification and question formulation* phase. In this phase, one needs to be able to develop and refine a range of questions to frame one's search and understand relevant health terms. In the second phase, *information search*, one has to possess appropriate searching skills, such as using proper keywords and correct spelling in search terms, especially when using search engines and databases. It is also crucial to understand how search engines work (i.e., how search results are derived, what the order of the search results means, how to use the snippets that are provided in the search results list to select websites, and how to determine which listings are ads on a search engine results page). One also has to limit reliance on surface characteristics, such as the design of a website or a book (a website or book that appears to have a lot of information or looks aesthetically pleasant does not necessarily mean it has good information) and language used (a website or book that utilizes jargon, the keywords that one used to conduct the search, or the word "information" does not necessarily indicate it will have good information). The next phase is *information comprehension*, whereby one needs to have the ability to read, comprehend, and recall the information (including textual, numerical, and visual content) one has located from the books and/or online resources.

To assess the credibility of health information (*information assessment* phase), one needs to be able to evaluate information for accuracy, evaluate how current the information is (e.g., when a website was last updated or when a book was published), and evaluate the creators of the source—for example, examine site sponsors or type of sites (.com,. gov,. edu, or. org) or the author of a book (practicing doctor, a celebrity doctor, a patient of a specific disease, etc.) to determine the believability of the person/organization providing the information. Such credibility perceptions tend to become generalized, so they must be frequently reexamined (e.g., the belief that a specific news agency always has credible health information needs continuous vetting). One also needs to evaluate the credibility of the medium (e.g., television, Internet, radio, social media, and book) and evaluate—not just accept without questioning—others' claims regarding the validity of a site, book, or other specific source of information. At this stage, one has to "make sense of information gathered from diverse sources by identifying misconceptions, main and supporting ideas, conflicting information, point of view, and biases" (American Association of School Librarians [AASL], 2009, p. 13) and conclude which sources/information are valid and accurate by using conscious strategies rather than simply using intuitive judgments or "rules of thumb." This phase is the most challenging segment of health information seeking and serves as a determinant of success (or lack thereof) in the information-seeking process. The following section "Sources of Health Information" further explains this phase.

The fifth phase is *information management*, whereby one has to organize information that has been gathered in some manner to ensure easy retrieval and use in the future. The last phase is *information use*, in which one will synthesize information found across various resources, draw conclusions, and locate the answer to one's original question and/or the content that fulfills the information need. This phase also often involves implementation, such as using the information to solve a health problem; make health-related decisions; identify and engage in behaviors that will help a person to avoid health risks; share the health information found with family members and friends who may benefit from it; and advocate more broadly for personal, family, or community health.

THE IMPORTANCE OF HEALTH LITERACY

The conception of health has moved from a passive view (someone is either well or ill) to one that is more active and process based (someone is working toward preventing or managing disease). Hence, the dominant focus has shifted from doctors and treatments to patients and prevention, resulting in the need to strengthen our ability and confidence (as patients and consumers of health care) to look for, assess, understand, manage, share, adapt, and use health-related information. An individual's health literacy level has been found to predict his or her health status better than age, race, educational attainment, employment status, and income level (National Network of Libraries of Medicine, 2013). Greater health literacy also enables individuals to better communicate with health-care providers such as doctors, nutritionists, and therapists, as they can pose more relevant, informed, and useful questions to health-care providers. Another added advantage of greater health literacy is better information-seeking skills, not only for health but also in other domains, such as completing assignments for school.

SOURCES OF HEALTH INFORMATION: THE GOOD, THE BAD, AND THE IN-BETWEEN

For generations, doctors, nurses, nutritionists, health coaches, and other health professionals have been the trusted sources of health information. In addition, researchers have found that young adults, when they have health-related questions, typically turn to a family member who has had firsthand experience with a health condition because of their family member's close proximity and because of their past experience with, and trust in, this individual. Expertise should be a core consideration when consulting a person, website, or book for health information. The credentials and background of the person or author and conflicting interests of the author (and his or her organization) must be checked and validated to ensure the likely credibility of the health information he or she is conveying. While books often have implied credibility because of the peer-review process involved, self-publishing has challenged this credibility, so qualifications of book authors should also be verified. When it comes to health information, currency of the source must also be examined. When examining health information/studies presented, pay attention to the exhaustiveness of research methods utilized to offer recommendations or conclusions. Small and nondiverse sample size is often—but not always—an indication of reduced credibility. Studies that confuse correlation with causation is another potential issue to watch for. Information seekers must also pay attention to the sponsors of the research studies. For example, if a study is sponsored by manufacturers of drug Y and the study recommends that drug Y is the best treatment to manage or cure a disease, this may indicate a lack of objectivity on the part of the researchers.

The Internet is rapidly becoming one of the main sources of health information. Online forums, news agencies, personal blogs, social media sites, pharmacy sites, and celebrity "doctors" are all offering medical and health information targeted at various types of people in regard to all types of diseases and symptoms. There are professional journalists, citizen journalists, hoaxers, and people paid to write fake health news on various sites that may appear to have a legitimate domain name and may even have authors who claim to have professional credentials, such as an MD. All these sites *may* offer useful information or information that appears to be useful and relevant; however, much of the information may be debatable and may fall into gray areas that require readers to discern credibility, reliability, and biases.

While broad recognition and acceptance of certain media, institutions, and people often serve as the most popular determining factors to assess credibility of health information among young people, keep in mind that there are legitimate Internet sites, databases, and books that publish health information and serve as sources of health information for doctors, other health sites, and members of the public. For example, MedlinePlus (https://medlineplus.gov) has trusted sources on over 975 diseases and conditions and presents the information in easy-to-understand language.

The chart here presents factors to consider when assessing credibility of health information. However, keep in mind that these factors function only as a guide and require continuous updating to keep abreast with the changes in the landscape of health information, information sources, and technologies.

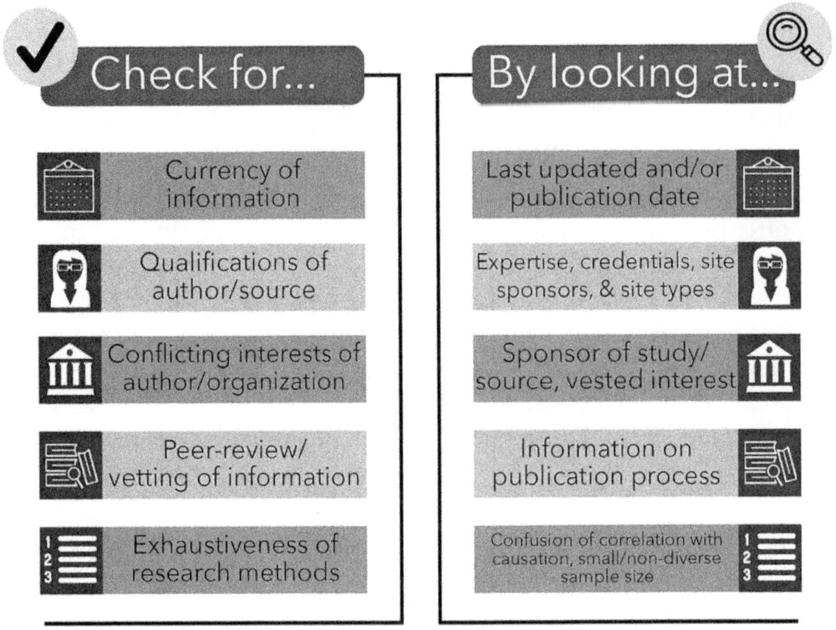

All images from flaticon.com

The chart can serve as a guide; however, approaching a librarian about how one can go about assessing the credibility of both print and online health information is far more effective than using generic checklist-type tools. While librarians are not health experts, they can apply and teach patrons strategies to determine the credibility of health information.

With the prevalence of fake sites and fake resources that appear to be legitimate, it is important to use the following health information assessment tips to verify health information that one has obtained (St. Jean et al., 2015, p. 151):

- **Don't assume you are right**: Even when you feel very sure about an answer, keep in mind that the answer may not be correct, and it is important to conduct (further) searches to validate the information.
- **Don't assume you are wrong**: You may actually have correct information, even if the information you encounter does not match—that is, you may be right and the resources that you have found may contain false information.
- **Take an open approach**: Maintain a critical stance by not including your preexisting beliefs as keywords (or letting them influence your

choice of keywords) in a search, as this may influence what it is possible to find out.

- **Verify, verify, and verify**: Information found, especially on the Internet, needs to be validated, no matter how the information appears on the site (i.e., regardless of the appearance of the site or the quantity of information that is included).

Health literacy comes with experience navigating health information. Professional sources of health information, such as doctors, health-care providers, and health databases, are still the best, but one also has the power to search for health information and then verify it by consulting with these trusted sources and by using the health information assessment tips and guide shared previously.

Mega Subramaniam, PhD
Associate Professor, College of Information Studies,
University of Maryland

REFERENCES AND FURTHER READING

American Association of School Librarians (AASL). (2009). *Standards for the 21st-century learner in action*. Chicago, IL: American Association of School Librarians.

Hilligoss, B., & Rieh, S.-Y. (2008). Developing a unifying framework of credibility assessment: Construct, heuristics, and interaction in context. *Information Processing & Management, 44*(4), 1467–1484.

Kuhlthau, C. C. (1988). Developing a model of the library search process: Cognitive and affective aspects. *Reference Quarterly, 28*(2), 232–242.

National Network of Libraries of Medicine (NNLM). (2013). Health literacy. Bethesda, MD: National Network of Libraries of Medicine. Retrieved from nnlm.gov/outreach/consumer/hlthlit.html.

Ratzan, S. C., & Parker, R. M. (2000). Introduction. In C. R. Selden, M. Zorn, S. C. Ratzan, & R. M. Parker (Eds.), *National Library of Medicine current bibliographies in medicine: Health literacy*. NLM Pub. No. CBM 2000-1. Bethesda, MD: National Institutes of Health, U.S. Department of Health and Human Services.

St. Jean, B., Subramaniam, M., Taylor, N. G., Follman, R., Kodama, C., & Casciotti, D. (2015). The influence of positive hypothesis testing on youths' online health-related information seeking. *New Library World, 116*(3/4), 136–154.

St. Jean, B., Taylor, N.G., Kodama, C., & Subramaniam, M. (February 2017). Assessing the health information source perceptions of tweens using card-sorting exercises. *Journal of Information Science*. Retrieved from http://journals.sagepub.com/doi/abs/10.1177/0165551516687728.

Subramaniam, M., St. Jean, B., Taylor, N.G., Kodama, C., Follman, R., & Casciotti, D. (2015). Bit by bit: Using design-based research to improve the health literacy of adolescents. *JMIR Research Protocols*, 4(2), paper e62. Retrieved from http://www.ncbi.nlm.nih.gov/pmc/articles/PMC4464334/.

Valenza, J. (2016, November 26). Truth, truthiness, and triangulation: A news literacy toolkit for a "post-truth" world [Web log]. Retrieved from http://blogs.slj.com/neverendingsearch/2016/11/26/truth-truthiness-triangulation-and-the-librarian-way-a-news-literacy-toolkit-for-a-post-truth-world/.

Common Misconceptions about Food Allergies and Sensitivities

1. EVERY NEGATIVE REACTION TO A FOOD IS AN ALLERGY

Not all adverse reactions that occur when eating a food are "true" allergic reactions. Only eight specific foods are associated with life-threatening reactions that involve the immune system. In fact, the majority of adverse food symptoms appear to be caused by food intolerances or sensitivities. Food intolerances and food sensitivities are much more subtle and may disguise themselves as chronic joint or gastrointestinal symptoms with no apparent trigger. Questions 1, 2, and 3 explore the differences among them in depth.

2. EXPERIENCING MILD REACTIONS TO A FOOD MEANS IT CAN STILL BE EATEN WITHOUT FEAR OF LIFE-THREATENING REACTIONS

Mild reactions to a food are usually a warning sign to avoid that food. Occasionally, a food can still be eaten if the individual is willing to live with minor symptoms. But, in general, food allergy reactions can progress from mild to life threatening in a matter of moments and at any time. In general, it is recommended that the food be avoided. Questions 18, 19, 20, and 21 discuss treatment for all adverse food reactions and emergency treatment methods.

3. ONCE A FOOD ALLERGY IS DIAGNOSED WHEN YOUNG, AN INDIVIDUAL IS ALLERGIC FOR THE REST OF HIS OR HER LIFE. CONVERSELY, IF AN INDIVIDUAL DOES NOT DEVELOP A FOOD ALLERGY WHEN YOUNG, HE OR SHE NEVER WILL

Children often outgrow most food allergies, although fish, peanut, shellfish, and tree nut allergies have a higher incidence of remaining a permanent affliction. As children become older they are often given food challenges, under medical supervision, to test if a food allergy has been outgrown. Adults may also develop food allergies as they age. But a greater percentage of negative reactions to food in adulthood are due to sensitivities or intolerances. Question 14 reviews adverse food reactions that are lifelong and temporary for both children and adults.

4. IF AN INDIVIDUAL HAS A FOOD ALLERGY, AN ANTI-HISTAMINE MEDICATION IS USUALLY ADEQUATE TREATMENT

As Question 21 highlights, emergency treatment for severe food reactions uses an injection of epinephrine with follow-up care in the emergency room. However, not all adverse food reactions are severe, and some can be managed with over-the-counter medications that contain anti-histamines. The mistake many food-sensitive individuals make is to assume mild reactions will never progress to life threatening. This assumption is a dangerous practice, and the investment in an Epi-Pen® or similar auto-injection device of epinephrine is an insurance policy that can mean the difference between life and death. Questions 18, 19, and 20 discuss the treatment options for all adverse food reactions.

5. FOOD BANS FOR PEANUT ALLERGIES IN SCHOOLS WILL PREVENT SEVERE ALLERGIC REACTIONS

Food bans in schools are a controversial debate. Pros and cons regarding the banning of highly allergenic foods in the school setting are discussed in depth in Question 22. It has been seen that food bans often provide a false sense of security and should never be relied on to protect an allergic individual from an adverse food reaction. Studies also show they are not as effective at protecting students as widely assumed.

QUESTIONS AND ANSWERS

Incidence and Diagnosis of Food Allergies, Intolerance, and Sensitivities

1. What is a food allergy?

Allergic reactions to a food will always involve the immune system. The job of the immune system is to protect the body from foreign invaders that have the potential to cause a serious illness or death. The human immune system is always in standby mode when a person is healthy. But if the body is invaded by something that it perceives as a threat to health, it switches on to actively fight against the threat. The immune system is bombarded daily with germs found in the air we breathe, through cuts or irritated skin, and by the foods we eat. When the immune system recognizes a threat, it responds by identifying the invader, marking it, attacking it, and destroying it. In the process of the attack, chemicals called inflammatory mediators (bradykinins, cytokines, histamine, leukotrienes, or prostaglandins) are released. Inflammatory mediators activate mast cells and leukocytes (white blood cells), which are involved in allergic reactions. These inflammatory mediators destroy the invader but can also produce allergy symptoms.

To understand how a food allergy occurs, it is important to understand the intricate workings of the human immune system. White blood cells, known as lymphocytes, eosinophils, and phagocytes, are in charge of protecting the body from threats. They are manufactured in many different areas of the body, which are then circulated to different organs via the bloodstream. Phagocytes destroy microorganisms, and lymphocytes target and assist in the destruction of foreign substances. There are two different types of lymphocytes, T cells and B cells. B cells form in the bone marrow and consist of mast cells and basophils. Mast cells travel to the respiratory tract, intestine, skin, and other body organs and are always on "patrol" and ready for action. Basophils circulate in the bloodstream and stay on alert for threats. T cells form in the thymus gland and alert B cells to make immunoglobulin antibodies, gather eosinophils in a specific location to fight the threat, or perform both. When the immune system is first exposed to a substance that may be harmful (bacteria, parasite, pathogen, or virus), it learns to recognize the substance by its molecular structure or antigen. Antigens are typically proteins but may be glycoproteins (proteins found in carbohydrate foods) or a molecule that is linked to a protein (e.g., a hormone or enzyme).

B cells are programmed to respond to specific shapes or structures, and they patrol looking for specific antigens. Once they identify a threatening antigen, T cells assist B cells by sending out signals for eosinophils to gather at a specific location. Immunoglobulin antibodies (Ig) are produced, which then attach themselves to the antigen so that the antigen is distinguished from healthy body cells that should not be attacked. When the eosinophils arrive at the directed area by the T cells, the eosinophils release chemicals that in turn destroy the invader and potentially cause inflammation and allergy symptoms.

There are five immunoglobulin antibodies that the immune system produces. These are IgG, IgA, IgE, IgM, and IgD. The IgG and IgM antibodies are the most commonly produced antibodies by the human immune system. Both attack bacteria, pathogens, and viruses that circulate in the bloodstream and lymph system, and IgM antibodies are usually produced first when an infection is present. IgA antibodies also attack bacteria, pathogens, and viruses but only in the gastrointestinal tract and breathing passages. IgE and IgD antibodies are specialty antibodies that are rarely produced. IgE antibodies are called up to fight parasitic infections but have been noted to increase during food allergy reactions. IgD antibody function remains unknown at this time. Reactions to an antigen that releases IgE antibodies are classified as IgE cell–mediated reactions, and these reactions occur within a few hours after exposure.

A food allergy is thought to occur when the immune system mistakenly identifies a specific food as a threat and overreacts by attacking it. IgE antibodies are usually directed at the protein component of a food, which in turn triggers an attack and allergic response that has the potential to be life threatening. It is estimated that 90 percent of food allergies worldwide are to eggs, cow's milk, legumes (peanuts, beans), sesame seeds, shellfish, soy, tree nuts, and wheat. However, other foods can produce an allergic reaction in some people.

Milk allergy is the most common food allergy in infants and young children under the age of three. Susceptible children tend to develop a milk allergy before they reach their first birthday, when their immune system identifies milk protein as harmful. Milk has two proteins, casein and whey, and a child can be allergic to one or the other or both. IgE antibodies are produced to neutralize the milk protein "allergen," and histamine and other chemicals are released, which in turn produces allergy symptoms ranging from anaphylaxis, abdominal cramps, colic, diarrhea, hives, rashes, runny nose, vomiting, watery eyes, or wheezing.

Allergies to eggs, legumes, sesame seeds, shellfish, soy, tree nuts, and wheat are also an allergic reaction to the protein component found in that food and are considered IgE-mediated reactions with similar symptoms to milk allergy. Egg, milk, and soy allergies are often outgrown. About 20–30 percent of children with sesame seed allergies tend to outgrow them. The likelihood of outgrowing peanut, shellfish, and tree nut allergies is rare, and these are often considered lifelong allergies. It is known that the earlier in age children experience a food allergy, the more likely they are to outgrow it. Approximately 27 percent of children outgrow their food allergy by the age of five.

It is still unclear why a person develops a food allergy. Some theories include genetic susceptibility. Children who develop food allergies are often allergic to pet dander, dust mites, grass pollen, and other environmental pollens and have other family members who have allergies. It is speculated that pollen proteins are very similar to the protein structure of a food, resulting in its misidentification as an allergen. It has also been speculated that being too clean, known as the "hygiene hypothesis," increases vulnerability for developing a food allergy as the immune system is bored and may be "looking for something to do."

There are some studies that show lack of exposure in the diet to peanuts when young may increase the risk for developing a peanut allergy. Another theory involves children born via caesarean section (C-section). These children are thought to have a weaker immune system, with a subsequent increase in susceptibility for infections and allergies, because they do not receive an essential transfer of bacteria that occurs during vaginal births. Recent studies find a connection between allergies and vaccinations because vaccinations alter the functioning of the immune system. Serum sickness, a common reaction to early vaccination methods, was identified by Dr. Clemens von Pirquet as an allergy in 1906.

2. What is a food intolerance?

Many people believe that all negative reactions to a food are a food allergy. But not all negative reactions to a food are a true allergic reaction. The distinction between a food intolerance and a food allergy is that true food allergies involve the immune system and can be life threatening. Food intolerances do not involve the immune system, are not usually life threatening, and tend to involve the digestive tract. They are also classified as either non-IgE-mediated or mixed IgE-mediated cell reactions, which means they may not produce IgE antibodies or some IgE antibodies are produced but symptoms can occur anywhere from hours to days after exposure.

The most common food intolerances are to fructose and lactose. Both involve difficulty digesting the sugar naturally present in these foods. Milk sugar, known as lactose, is found in dairy foods. Fructose sugar is found in fruits, fruit juice, some vegetables, and honey. In general, a food intolerance is usually caused by the absence or deficiency of a digestive enzyme in the gastrointestinal tract. The gastrointestinal tract and different organs, such as the liver, pancreas, and gall bladder, normally produce digestive enzymes. These enzymes are necessary for the proper digestion of foods. The body produces and uses thousands of enzymes daily to ensure proper biochemical reactions that are necessary for health occur. To better understand this process in breaking down the foods we eat, it is necessary to understand the digestion of foods.

The basic process of digesting foods involves six steps.

1. Chewing foods releases the first digestive enzyme, salivary amylase, in the mouth. Salivary amylase breaks down starchy foods, partially digesting the carbohydrates found in starches before the food moves into the stomach.
2. As the food moves into the stomach, the parietal cells of the stomach release acids (e.g., hydrochloric acid), enzymes, and pancreatic amylase (which is different from salivary amylase). Pancreatic amylase differs from salivary amylase because it is released by the pancreas and is an enzyme that dissolves complex carbohydrates, which take longer to digest, in the stomach and small intestine. These substances all

continue to further break down this partially digested food mass, now called chyme, into small components that the body can absorb and use.

3. Chyme remains in the stomach for about an hour and is then propelled into the duodenum, which is the upper part of the small intestine. In the duodenum the hormone secretin is released to further digest the chyme.
4. The release of secretin signals the pancreas to release hormones, bicarbonate, bile, and other enzymes to continue the digestion process.
5. Pancreatic enzymes include amylase, lipase, proteases, and peptidases. Each enzyme has a specific function and type of food that it breaks down into usable forms of energy. Amylase breaks down starchy foods. Proteases and peptidases break down protein foods. Lipases break down fatty foods.
6. Bicarbonate changes the acidity of chyme to make it more alkaline, which allows the enzymes to continue to break down food. An alkaline environment also destroys any potentially harmful bacteria that are capable of living in an acidic environment.

In addition to the basic digestive enzymes of amylase, proteases, and lipase, specialty enzymes are released to digest specific foods. For instance, the enzyme lactase is released to break down the sugar lactose present in milk and milk-based foods. Typical symptoms of lactose intolerance include abdominal pain or stomachache, bloating, constipation, cough, diarrhea, gas, headaches or migraines, hives, irritable bowel, and runny nose.

But food intolerances do not always involve digestive enzymes. Fructose is one example. In most people fructose is absorbed when passing through the small intestine directly into the bloodstream without any need for a digestive enzyme. However, fructose intolerance can be the result of an inability to absorb fructose properly or because of an inherited gene.

There are two types of fructose intolerance: hereditary fructose intolerance (HFI) and fructose malabsorption. HFI is due to a deficiency of the enzyme aldolase B, which is produced by the liver. Fructose malabsorption differs from HFI and occurs when fructose cannot pass through the small intestinal wall, resulting in a buildup of it in the intestine, which then produces typical symptoms of abdominal cramps, bloating, gas, diarrhea or constipation, dizziness, fatigue, nausea, reflux or heartburn, severe hypoglycemia, and stomachache.

For any other food intolerance, symptoms are also similar to those listed for both lactose and fructose intolerances. Treatment for all food intolerances includes strictly avoiding the food in the daily diet and using digestive enzymes or short-term antibiotics as indicated. A medical professional should always evaluate anyone with a food intolerance.

3. What is a food sensitivity?

Many medical professionals and food allergy organizations use the term "food sensitivity," also known as "food hypersensitivity," as a comprehensive term to describe both food allergies and intolerances. But food sensitivity reactions differ from food allergies and food intolerances. These negative reactions sometimes involve the immune system but may also affect the brain, gastrointestinal system, joints, skin, and respiratory tract. Food sensitivities tend to be much more complicated to diagnose because symptoms often seem unrelated to a specific food or may occur when specific foods are eaten together. Symptoms can also occur days and weeks after eating the suspected food. Food sensitivity reactions often take years to properly diagnose and may be debilitating for some and life threatening for others.

Hypersensitivity reactions are classified into Type I, Type II, Type III, and Type IV categories. Type I hypersensitivity reactions are immediate reactions to a trigger. IgE antibodies, mast cells, and basophils are all activated and release inflammatory mediators (e.g., histamine) in response to an antigen. Type I include food allergy reactions with anaphylaxis as a common symptom. Type II hypersensitivity reactions activate IgM and IgG antibodies that target and destroy specific body tissues. These reactions are not involved in food reactions and can cause specific diseases such as anemia, Graves' disease, and Goodpasture syndrome. Type III hypersensitivity reactions produce antibodies that cause inflammation. These reactions affect the immune system, causing tissue damage. Reactions classified as Type III hypersensitivity are serum sickness, lupus, IgA nephropathy, and Arthus reactions from vaccines. Type IV hypersensitivity reactions are cell mediated and are delayed reactions in which T cell lymphocytes, rather than antibodies, are activated. Examples of Type IV hypersensitivity include contact dermatitis (from poison ivy, cosmetics, rubber gloves), drug reactions, and multiple sclerosis. Type IV hypersensitivity is also implicated in celiac disease (CD) and food-induced enterocolitis. It is thought that food sensitivities are a Type IV hypersensitivity.

Food sensitivities appear intertwined with the autoimmune response of the body. A disease is classified as an autoimmune disorder when the body's immune system attacks and destroys healthy body cells by mistake. Currently there are over 80 known autoimmune diseases. Autoimmune diseases involve the T cells and B cells of the immune system. These lymphocytes can, when something goes awry, become activated to attack normal cells for destruction, causing symptoms. An autoimmune disease can destroy body tissue, cause abnormal growths, and change the function of an organ as well as affect blood vessels and red blood cells, connective tissue, muscles and joints, endocrine glands, and skin.

The autoimmune disease process involving foods is considered an abnormal immune reaction to a food, food additive, or food chemical. But food sensitivity reactions don't always involve an autoimmune process. Sometimes toxins that cause food poisoning or a toxic amount of a naturally occurring chemical, such as histamine, found in a food can elicit food sensitivity symptoms. The most well-known and medically recognized abnormal reactions to food include the following:

- Gluten-sensitive enteropathy, also known as celiac sprue or CD
- Food-dependent, exercise-induced anaphylaxis (FDEIA)
- Allergic eosinophilic gastroenteritis
- Food protein-induced enterocolitis syndrome
- Food protein-induced proctocolitis
- Oral allergy syndrome
- Sulfite-induced asthma
- Leaky gut

Gluten-sensitive enteropathy, also known as celiac sprue, is classified as a gluten intolerance or wheat allergy. However, it is neither a true intolerance nor a true allergy. It is an abnormal response by the immune system to gluten and considered an autoimmune disease. Autoimmune diseases will trigger either an abnormally low or overactive response by the immune system. When it is overactive, the body begins to attack and destroy its own tissues. It is still not clear exactly why the body reacts this way. But gluten-sensitive enteropathy typically manifests itself in individuals who have a genetic predisposition, eat gluten-containing foods in their diet, and may also be experiencing stress or a trauma in their life or have a viral infection. Wheat allergy is distinct from celiac sprue and non-celiac gluten sensitivity because it is a true allergy reaction with symptoms that are usually immediate and life threatening. CD symptoms are chronic and debilitating over time.

CD is a genetic, autoimmune disorder. At-risk individuals usually carry either the *HLA DQ2* or *DQ8* genes or both. Although an estimated 40 percent of the population has these genes, it does not always indicate they will develop CD. However, individuals with a parent, sibling, or child who is diagnosed with CD will be predisposed to develop CD themselves if they carry these genes. Therefore, family members are usually tested for these genes and monitored for CD symptoms.

Treatment for CD requires a strict gluten-free diet for life. Gluten is a protein found in wheat and barley and can be toxic to those with CD. When gluten-sensitive individuals eat gluten, the finger-like ridges in the walls (mucosa) of the small intestine become flattened and severely damaged. When this happens, the mucosa is unable to absorb food nutrients properly, and intestinal permeability is increased. The result is severe and life-threatening symptoms due to malabsorption of nutrients and substances crossing into the bloodstream that would normally be prevented from doing so. Individuals experiencing severe symptoms will be screened using blood tests that check for CD antibodies. The most common blood test ordered is a tissue transglutaminase (tTG) antibody-IgA antibody test (tTg-IgA). A tTg-IgA antibody test measures specific antibodies that are usually elevated when someone has CD. For accurate results, the individual must be eating foods with gluten and not following a gluten-free diet. If this test is positive, then the individual will undergo a biopsy of the small intestine to confirm a CD diagnosis. Once gluten is removed from the diet, the small intestine mucosa begins to heal and nutrients are then absorbed normally, and the intestinal barrier heals, resulting in improved health and resolution of symptoms.

But gluten-sensitive individuals may also be classified as having non-celiac gluten sensitivity (NCGS). Symptoms of NCGS are similar to those with CD. Although tTg-IgA antibody tests and small intestine biopsy results are negative for these individuals, there are some who experience symptoms of bloating, gas, abdominal pain, diarrhea or constipation, nausea, headache, brain fog, joint pain, fatigue, or numbness in legs, arms, and fingers after eating gluten-containing foods. It has been generally recognized that NCGS is less severe than CD because there is minimal intestinal damage. Elimination of gluten from the diet usually allows the intestine to heal and symptoms to improve or resolve.

FDEIA is a rare food sensitivity that occurs only if an individual eats a specific food and exercises within a one- to four-hour period before or after eating it. The symptoms are usually mild but can progress to be life threatening. If the food is eaten at any other time without exercise, symptoms do not occur. Alcohol, apples, celery, dairy, egg, fish, fruit, legumes, milk, nuts, shellfish, and wheat are the most common triggers of FDEIA, but any food combined with exercise can trigger it. Females are more susceptible than males, and it tends to occur more often in people between the ages of 25 and 35 years, who also have asthma and seasonal allergies or take aspirin or non-steroidal anti-inflammatory drugs. Exercising in warm and humid temperatures appears to trigger symptoms as well. Susceptible women tend to experience symptoms of FDEIA during menstruation, indicating a possible hormonal connection.

While it is still unclear exactly why FDEIA reactions occur, there appears to be a connection between specific insoluble proteins, such as gluten, and a normal increase in intestinal absorption of food proteins that occurs during exercise when food proteins have not yet been completely digested. Individuals with a family history of FDEIA appear to be more susceptible, indicating a possible genetic predisposition.

Allergic eosinophilic gastroenteritis occurs when there is an overabundance of eosinophils in the lining of the digestive tract. Eosinophils are one type of white blood cell produced by the immune system when there is an infection or inflammation. Eosinophil levels can be elevated if an individual has parasitic or fungal infections, adrenal disease, skin disorders, toxin exposure, autoimmune or endocrine disorders, or tumors.

While rare, allergic eosinophilic gastroenteritis occurs when an excessive number of eosinophils accumulate in the gastrointestinal system in response to an antigen, which interferes with the normal function of the gastrointestinal tract. Symptoms include abdominal pain, bloody diarrhea, fatigue, malnutrition, nausea, vomiting, and weight loss.

Food protein–induced enterocolitis syndrome (FPIES) is usually diagnosed in infants and children, but cases have been reported in adults. FPIES is a non-IgE-mediated food reaction that affects the gastrointestinal system and does not involve an immune system release of antibodies. However, it does appear to involve T cells, which attack perceived harmful antigens. T cells are lymphocytes that are produced in the thymus gland when an antigen is identified. T cells then alert B cells, another lymphocyte produced when an antigen is identified, to make immunoglobulin antibodies, gather eosinophils in a specific location to fight the threat, or perform both.

Symptoms are usually severe and include severe and repetitive vomiting and diarrhea, lethargy, poor growth, and pale appearance. The most common trigger foods are chicken, eggs, cow's milk, nuts, peanuts, rice, soy, turkey, and wheat. Breastfed babies rarely develop FPIES, but babies on milk or soy-based formulas are more susceptible. It is speculated that an immature gastrointestinal system that is not yet able to properly digest milk or soy may trigger symptoms. Shellfish is the most common trigger food for susceptible adults. However, any food may trigger symptoms of FPIES. Treatment includes avoiding the trigger food in the diet. Young children with FPIES tend to outgrow their food sensitivity.

Food protein–induced proctocolitis (FPIPC), also known as allergic or eosinophilic proctocolitis or protein intolerance, typically occurs within the first few months of a susceptible infant's life. It is considered an allergy, rather than sensitivity, because of an abnormal response to a food protein. Because of this it is thought to be a transient colitis for unknown reasons. Traditional allergy testing has been a useful diagnostic method for FPIPC, and diagnosis is usually made using a sigmoidoscopy examination and a rectal mucosal biopsy of the large intestine.

FPIPC is triggered most often by cow's milk or soy protein and is usually outgrown by one to three years of age. However, corn and eggs may also cause symptoms, and any food protein may trigger symptoms. It is theorized that the immature gastrointestinal system of the infant is unable to distinguish between good and bad proteins, thus inflaming the lower part of the intestines. Symptoms include bloody, watery, or green bowel movements, a very fussy baby, discomfort after eating, poor sleep, or crying all day and night. An estimated 25 percent of babies develop FPIPC, and, while no specific cause has yet been discovered, it is known the majority of affected babies are born into a family that has food allergies. Treatment involves avoiding all trigger foods.

Oral allergy syndrome is an allergic reaction to a protein found in environmental pollens. Some raw fruits and vegetables have the same protein structure that is also found in tree and plant pollens. This in turn triggers the body to "recognize" it as a pollen allergen to be attacked. However, when the trigger food is cooked, the protein component of the food is broken down (denatured), and, in general, the individual is often able to eat the food without experiencing symptoms.

Oral allergy syndrome is not considered a true allergy because diagnosis is often made based on reported symptoms. Skin prick tests will often be positive, but oral food challenges are the usual diagnostic method used to confirm oral allergy syndrome. Symptoms include itchy or scratchy mouth, swelling of the lips, mouth, tongue, and throat. Itchy ears have also been reported. Treatment involves avoiding the suspected foods, which vary depending on the pollen allergy.

Sulfite-induced asthma is an adverse reaction to sulfites found in foods or medications. Sulfites are a preservative added to some foods to prevent them from spoiling, thus extending their shelf life. They are specifically prohibited in some foods, such as meat, because they will remove vitamins from the food making it less nutritious. Sulfites are most commonly added to some alcoholic drinks, baked goods, shredded coconut, condiments, fruits, canned or bottled fruit and vegetables, gelatin and pudding or filling mixes, dried fruits and snacks, drink mixes, grains, jams and preserves, molasses, pastries, soup mixes, and vegetables. But they can also occur naturally in foods, such as broccoli, cabbage, cauliflower, chives, eggs, garlic, kale, leeks, onions, peanuts, black tea, vinegar, and other fermented foods. Sulfites may also be found in some prescription medications. Symptoms of sulfite-induced asthma include anaphylaxis, asthma attacks or difficulty breathing, diarrhea, difficulty swallowing, dizziness, hives, itchiness, low blood pressure, upset stomach, and vomiting. Treatment includes avoiding all foods with added or naturally occurring sulfites and carrying an EpiPen.

Leaky gut syndrome, also called increased intestinal permeability, is a recently identified food-related diagnosis that is gaining more attention but still remains controversial within the medical community. Before medical diagnostic methods improved, early physicians often believed the root of certain ailments originated in the intestines. In recent years the digestive tract has been discovered to play a larger role in immunity and health than previously realized. The stomach and gastrointestinal tract are responsible for breaking down food into nutrients that are used for energy, hormone, enzyme, vitamin production, immune defense, and different biochemical reactions that occur within the body to keep it running and healthy.

Both the stomach and the intestinal tract have a protective lining made up of epithelial cells. Epithelial cells are everywhere in our bodies and are a safety shield between the inside of the body and the outside world. This lining protects the gastrointestinal tract from strong digestive acids used to break down and extract nutrients from food and from potentially dangerous toxins and microorganisms. In the small intestine, epithelial cells are packed tightly together to prevent undigested food particles or other substances from passing through the small intestine into the bloodstream. But sometimes a disease, such Crohn's disease, or a food sensitivity can damage these epithelial cells. Dysbiosis, which is an imbalance of harmful and beneficial microorganisms that live normally in the gastrointestinal tract (microbiome), may also trigger a leaky gut. Antibiotic medications can disrupt this finally balanced microbiome. The result can be an overabundance of harmful bacteria in relation to beneficial bacteria living in the gastrointestinal tract and an increase in systemic inflammation.

"Sensitivity" reactions appear to cause the gastrointestinal epithelial cells' normally tight junctions to loosen up, creating "holes," which increase permeability and allow undigested foods or substances to escape through this barrier into the bloodstream. This in turn appears to trigger symptoms, illness, and some chronic diseases. This increased intestinal permeability has been called "leaky gut syndrome." It is theorized that when undigested food particles escape into the bloodstream, the body's immune system is activated causing a myriad of symptoms. It has been discovered that immune cells, which contain the white blood cell neutrophil elastase, increase when mast cell mediators (e.g., tryptase and histamine) increase in the colon. Mast cell mediators are chemicals produced during an allergic reaction by the immune system. An increase in elastase appears to cause tissue damage, which may in turn increase intestinal permeability. Symptoms vary from person to person and are thought to include food allergies, acne, asthma, autism, autoimmune diseases (type I diabetes, lupus, multiple sclerosis), bloating, CD, Crohn's disease, chronic fatigue syndrome, eczema and psoriasis, fibromyalgia, inflammatory bowel disease, irritable bowel syndrome, rheumatoid arthritis, and systemic inflammatory response syndrome. However, research studies have yet to verify a connection between leaky gut syndrome and these medical conditions.

4. What are the signs and symptoms of a food allergy?

Symptoms of a food allergy range from minor, such as hives, to life-threatening anaphylaxis, and they vary from person to person. Food allergy symptoms typically occur within minutes after eating a suspected food but can take up to 10–15 minutes or a few hours to appear. Symptoms often completely disappear within one to two hours after eating a trigger food.

The most severe and life-threatening symptoms of a food allergy, known as acute symptoms, affect the cardiovascular and respiratory systems, impairing blood circulation and the ability to breathe. Anaphylaxis is the most severe symptom and is an acute hypersensitivity reaction to a food protein that causes the immune system to release a large quantity of chemicals to counteract it. This cascade of chemicals causes blood pressure to drop suddenly and narrows airways, significantly decreasing the ability of the cardiovascular and respiratory systems to function with often fatal results. Frequently reported symptoms include asthma, anaphylactic shock, difficulty or inability to breathe, chills, fainting, irregular heartbeat, low blood pressure, pale or bluish skin tone, feeling of panic, sense of doom, sudden weakness, tight feeling in the chest, or wheezing.

Chronic symptoms of a food allergy are not usually life threatening and can affect many different body systems. Frequently the gastrointestinal system is affected because foods are digested in this system. A trigger allergenic food will irritate the intestinal lining, causing a constant inflammation within the gastrointestinal tract. Frequently reported symptoms affecting the intestinal tract include abdominal pain or cramps; diarrhea; nausea; lip, mouth, or tongue swelling; and vomiting. Chronic exposure to allergenic foods may also manifest as skin symptoms due to systemic body inflammation with symptoms of eczema and hives, itching or swelling of the face, itchy rash, and generalized swelling. Lungs and airways may have an accumulation of eosinophils along bronchial passage ways causing symptoms of cough, hoarse voice, runny nose, and throat swelling.

5. What are the signs and symptoms of food intolerance?

Symptoms of food intolerance most frequently involve the gastrointestinal tract and often begin anywhere from within a few minutes to a few hours after eating a trigger food. Symptoms vary from person to person, but the most frequently reported symptoms include abdominal pain or stomachache, bloating, constipation or diarrhea, cough, gas, headaches or migraines, hives, irritable bowel, and runny nose.

Food intolerances are typically caused by an absent or inadequate amount of a digestive enzyme that is necessary to fully digest food passing through the gastrointestinal tract. Because of a lack or inadequate supply of a digestive enzyme, food is only partially digested as it passes through the digestive system. As a result, these partially digested foods are broken down using the process of fermentation. Fermentation is a process in which food is broken down into easily digestible forms that can be used by the bacteria found in the gastrointestinal tract. However, a by-product of fermentation is the production of hydrogen sulfide, nitric oxide, ammonia, and methane. This gas production in the gut accumulates and causes the symptoms of abdominal pain, bloating, constipation, passing gas, or diarrhea.

Fermentation can also increase the amount of amines in the intestines. Amines are substances created by bacteria that break down protein into amino acids. Histamine and tyramine are the two amines most people are intolerant to. When amines accumulate in the intestine, they can produce symptoms that include cough, hives, itching, rash, stomachache or irritable bowel, mental confusion, migraines or headaches, runny nose, and vomiting.

One exception is hereditary fructose intolerance, which occurs due to the lack of the enzyme aldolase B, which is produced by the liver. Individuals with hereditary fructose intolerance are unable to digest fructose. This, in turn, causes fructose to build up in the intestine, producing the same symptoms as other intolerances. But in hereditary fructose intolerance fructose is also absorbed into the bloodstream, where it does not undergo conversion to glucose. The result is severe hypoglycemia with fatal results if left untreated.

6. What are the signs and symptoms of food sensitivity?

As with food intolerances, symptoms vary from person to person and include all the same symptoms that can occur with food allergies and intolerances. However, many unrelated symptoms associated with chronic diseases or conditions are also thought to indicate a food sensitivity reaction. These include joint pain, arthritis, inflammatory bowel disease, nutritional deficiencies, autism, "brain fog" or memory loss, and numerous environmental allergies.

Medically recognized food sensitivities include gluten-sensitive enteropathy, non-celiac gluten sensitivity, food-dependent, exercise-induced anaphylaxis, allergic eosinophilic gastroenteritis, food protein–induced enterocolitis syndrome, food protein–induced proctocolitis, oral allergy syndrome symptoms, sulfite-induced asthma, and leaky gut. Each of these sensitivities is distinguished by specific symptoms.

Frequently reported symptoms of gluten-sensitive enteropathy, an autoimmune disease also known as celiac sprue, include abdominal bloating and frequent passing of gas, diarrhea, and weight loss. Eating gluten foods in the diet causes damage to small intestine mucosa in susceptible individuals. This, in turn, reduces the ability to digest and absorb nutrients from food, resulting in nutrient deficiencies and weight loss. Partially digested food in the intestinal tract also undergoes fermentation, which produces bloating, passing of gas, and diarrhea symptoms.

Non-celiac gluten sensitivity, while not classified as an autoimmune disease, is also caused by a gluten sensitivity with small intestine damage. Symptoms are similar to gluten-sensitive enteropathy but also include brain fog; fatigue; headache; joint pain; nausea; and numbness in arms, fingers, and legs. These symptoms are thought to result from a buildup of gluten by-products in the system from undigested gluten that affects different body systems.

Food-dependent, exercise-induced anaphylaxis symptoms occur only if an individual eats a trigger food and exercises. If the food is eaten but the individual does not exercise, then symptoms do not usually occur. Symptoms typically occur anywhere from one to four hours before or after the trigger food is eaten and include itchy or reddened skin, swelling, hives, and possible progression to anaphylaxis. It is thought undigested proteins that cross into the bloodstream can cause symptoms that affect the cardiovascular, gastrointestinal, and respiratory systems.

Allergic eosinophilic gastroenteritis occurs when there is a buildup of eosinophils, which are white blood cells, along the gastrointestinal tract. Because there is an excess number of eosinophils in the digestive tract, which reduces the ability of the gastrointestinal tract to digest foods and absorb nutrients, typical symptoms reported are nausea and vomiting after eating, chronic abdominal pain, diarrhea, growth delays in children, and weight loss in adults.

Food protein–induced enterocolitis syndrome (FPIES) affects babies and children in the majority of cases reported. However, adults can also develop FPIES. Symptoms can occur anywhere from one to six hours after ingesting the trigger food, and the first typical sign of FPIES is severe vomiting or diarrhea after eating the suspected food. Other reported symptoms are dehydration, lethargy, low blood pressure, poor growth, and pale or blue skin appearance. Trigger foods appear to inflame and irritate the gastrointestinal tract causing damage and an inability to digest foods and absorb nutrients properly. Adult symptoms are the same.

Food protein–induced proctocolitis is diagnosed only in infants and commonly occurs during the first few months of life. The first sign of food protein–induced proctocolitis is bright red blood after a bowel movement. It is thought to be caused by an inability to digest foods, causing an inflamed gastrointestinal tract. Other reported symptoms include green or watery bowel movements, discomfort after eating, fussiness, poor sleep, and crying all day and night.

A protein found in environmental pollens that is also found in most fruits and vegetables causes oral allergy syndrome. Because the immune system attacks foreign pollens to protect itself, symptoms occur because the food protein structure is closely similar to the pollen protein. Typical symptoms include an itching or burning sensation in the mouth, lips, ear canal, or throat. Swelling of lips, tongue, and uvula; throat tightness; vomiting; diarrhea; indigestion; and cramps may also occur. Severe symptoms are rare, and if the food is cooked, symptoms usually do not occur.

Sulfite-induced asthma symptoms occur because of an adverse reaction to added and naturally occurring sulfites found in foods. The respiratory system is typically affected, causing asthma symptoms of difficulty swallowing or breathing, feeling faint, or loss of consciousness. But other reported symptoms include abdominal pain, cramping, diarrhea, nausea, and vomiting. Skin symptoms of hives, itching, rashes, and localized swelling can also occur. The cardiovascular system may also be affected, and symptoms include headache, chest pain, and changes in body temperature or heart rate. Reactions to sulfites are often life threatening.

A gastrointestinal tract that is damaged allows undigested foods, bacteria, and toxins into the bloodstream, causing a leaky gut. This, in turn, allows these substances to be circulated throughout the body, affecting many different body systems. Typically reported symptoms vary from person to person and include asthma, autism, autoimmune diseases, bloating and gas, brain fog, constipation, diarrhea, difficulty digesting foods, eczema and psoriasis, chemical or environmental allergies, excess fatigue, headaches, poor immunity, inflammatory bowel disease, joint pain, memory loss, nutritional deficiencies, rashes, rheumatoid arthritis, runny nose, vitamin and mineral deficiencies, and systemic inflammatory response syndrome.

7. How are food allergies diagnosed?

The accurate diagnosis of food allergies can be challenging because current testing methods are not always reliable. The first step toward an accurate diagnosis is an assessment by a trained allergist. An allergist is a medical doctor who specializes in the diagnosis and treatment of all types of allergies. An allergist will perform a physical examination and medical history review, ordering skin tests and blood tests if indicated. There are four different testing methods used to confirm a food allergy diagnosis. They are the skin prick test, blood testing, oral food challenge, and trial elimination diet.

The skin prick test, also called scratch testing, is usually the first test completed because it produces immediate results, is inexpensive, and is easily done in the doctors' office. A drop of solution containing different common food allergens is placed onto the skin of the forearm or back. Sometimes fresh fruits or vegetables will be rubbed on the skin instead of the solution. A small plastic needle is then used to gently scratch the skin, allowing a small amount of the solution to enter the skin just below the surface. If a raised white bump surrounded by a small circle of itchy red skin occurs within 30 minutes, the test indicates a positive reaction and an allergy to that particular food. If there is no skin reaction, the test is considered negative. In general, negative results are thought to be almost always accurate. However, positive skin prick test results have a 50–60 percent accuracy rate. "False"-positive results are very common. This is thought to occur because the digestive tract breaks down food proteins into small molecules, which the body may be unable to detect.

Since these tests do not mimic the digestive process, food proteins are larger when they interact with the skin or blood, making it easier for IgE antibodies to "see." This in turn then shows sensitivity to a food that may be inaccurate. Therefore, skin prick tests are not always a reliable method of food allergy diagnosis, and further testing is recommended if there is a positive result to the skin prick test.

A blood test will then be ordered if skin prick testing is positive and is frequently used to detect food allergies. In 1903 the pediatrician Clemens von Piquet was the first to identify elevated IgE blood levels during an allergic reaction. Blood tests measure the presence of immunoglobulin E (IgE) antibody production in the bloodstream in response to specific foods. Allergy blood tests used in the past were called radioallergosorbent (RAST) tests because they used a radioactive substance to identify IgE. New testing methods that identify IgE have replaced the RAST but no longer use any materials that are radioactive.

Prior to the day of the test, any suspected food is avoided in the diet by the patient until the day of the test. On the day of the test, blood is taken from the individual and put into a test tube. Depending on the lab, the protein from the suspected food or foods will be placed onto a solid item, such as a paper disk, gel matrix, or plastic bead. This item will then be placed into the test tube of blood. If IgE antibodies are present in the blood, they will attach themselves to the protein. The test tube is processed so that only the IgE antibodies are left in the tube attached to the protein. The IgE levels are then measured. Elevated numbers of IgE antibodies indicate a positive allergy to the food tested.

However, this blood test also has an accuracy rate similar to skin prick tests. About 50–60 percent of the time the test may show a positive reaction to a food protein even though the person does not experience symptoms when he or she eats that particular food. Blood tests are very sensitive, but they are not very specific, meaning they are often positive when there is no allergy. It is also speculated that results may be false positive in response to the presence of undigested food proteins or that the body is detecting the same proteins found in many different foods. For example, peanuts and chic peas are both legumes and have the same protein molecule. A person may be allergic to peanuts but not chic peas, even though they are both legumes. But even though blood tests are not the most accurate predictor of a food allergy, they are one helpful tool for the allergist in identifying a potential food allergy.

If skin prick and blood tests do not clearly indicate an allergy, an oral food challenge test may then be recommended. It is used infrequently, however, because of the potential risk for a serious and life-threatening allergic reaction. This test should always be administered in a hospital or medical facility where emergency care is available in the event of a life-threatening reaction. In general, however, it is safe when administered under the direction of an experienced allergist.

During an oral food challenge, the individual eats very small and measured amounts of the suspected allergenic food in a powder form. The food is presented in a powdered form to minimize bias toward the food by the patient and doctor. If there is no reaction over a measured amount of time, continued small amounts are eaten until a reaction does occur. Generally mild symptoms, like hives or flushing, will occur if the individual is allergic. Rarely do severe reactions occur. A positive reaction is usually accurate and will confirm a food allergy.

There are three kinds of oral food challenges an allergist can use: double-blind, placebo-controlled food challenge, single-blind food challenge, and open blind food challenge. In the double-blind, placebo-controlled food challenge, which is considered the "gold standard" and most accurate method for food allergy diagnosis, the individual receives increasing doses of suspected foods or a placebo. However, neither the doctor nor the individual knows what the powdered food is. This prevents the individual from having an "allergic reaction" just from looking at the food, which can happen when an association is made between a food and symptoms. This oral challenge ensures the results are objective. In the single-blind food challenge, only the allergist knows what foods are being tested. In the open blind food challenge, both the allergist and individual know the food or foods being tested.

The food elimination diet may also be used. This test is another diagnostic tool used to confirm a food allergy diagnosis. A specific diet plan that removes all suspected foods is eaten for a two- to four-week period. Symptoms are monitored during this time. If they disappear, it is usually concluded that the eliminated food was the cause of symptoms. Often, after the diet has concluded, one food will be reintroduced into the diet and return of symptoms monitored. If symptoms reoccur, then it is usually recommended that that food be eliminated permanently from the diet. After a two- to three-day period of eating the reintroduced food, another food will be reintroduced, and the preceding procedure will be repeated until all foods are reintroduced into the diet and a determination will be made regarding sensitivity to it.

A typical elimination diet removes eggs, fish, milk, peanuts, shellfish, soy, tree nuts, and wheat from the diet for a period of two to four weeks because these foods are the most common food allergens that elicit an allergic response by the majority of susceptible individuals. However, other foods may be eliminated if indicated. Only low allergenic foods (apples, beef, berries, broccoli, chicken, corn, rice, string beans, and sweet potatoes) are eaten during this time until eliminated foods are reintroduced one at a time.

There are also other testing methods used to "diagnose" food allergies, but most of these tests are not used or recommended by allergists because very little evidence has been found that proves their accuracy. These include muscle testing, cytotoxicity testing, electrodermal tests, natural elimination of allergy treatment (NEAT) and Nambrudipad's Allergy Elimination Technique (NAET), IgG and IgG4 testing, hair analysis, and pulse testing.

Muscle testing, also known as applied kinesiology, is an alternative medicine method used to test for food allergies and sensitivities. Some acupuncturists, chiropractors, and naturopathic physicians administer this test while the patient holds a vial of the suspected allergen in front of specific areas of the body. As the patient holds the vial with one arm, the practitioner faces the patient and lifts the opposite arm out to the side, testing the muscles of that arm by applying pressure on it. It is assumed that the patient has a specific food allergy if arm muscle weakness occurs during the test. Some practitioners may also vary the test by adding magnets. However, there is no medical evidence that this test method is accurate, and it is considered unreliable.

Cytotoxicity testing, also called Bryan's Test, involves assessing a patient's white blood cells, which are prepared in a suspension solution, after they are mixed with a dried food extract solution. This mixture is placed onto a microscope slide and examined after 10 minutes. It is reexamined in 30-minute intervals up to two hours later. The patient is deemed allergic or sensitive if the white blood cells disintegrate or become distorted. The American Academy of Allergy and the Food and Drug Administration have determined this test is ineffective and has no scientific basis proving its accuracy.

The electrodermal test (Vega testing) applies a small amount of direct electric current to a specific skin point to determine if the patient has a food allergy or sensitivity. It is thought that offending allergens can generate measurable electric changes at specific acupuncture points. This test has no evidence supporting it and has usually resulted in many false-positive results. It is not a recommended test for food allergy diagnosis.

NEAT and NAET belong in the category of energy medicine. Energy medicine is one branch of alternative medicine that harnesses the natural energy system of the body. Electronic devices are used to measure body energy currents and therapies applied that are considered to bring the body's energy back into balance. These therapies include acupuncture, massage, yoga, and various other alternative methods. NEAT and NAET protocols involve measuring how well energy flows at specific acupuncture sites with a blunt probe. If the electrical conduction is impaired or suboptimal at these points, then sensitivities are diagnosed. This method also includes energy balance treatments using electrical stimulation and homeopathic treatments to reduce allergies and sensitivities. No scientific studies support the accuracy of the NEAT and NAET tests, and this testing method is not recommended as a diagnostic tool.

IgG and IgG4 testing is a bit more controversial, with a number of dietitians and naturopathic doctors convinced of its validity as a food allergen testing tool. Also known as Mediator Release Test (MRT) and antigen leukocyte cellular antibody test (ALCAT), these tests are used primarily to identify food sensitivities. Both show promise in diagnosing food sensitivities but are controversial among the medical community. The MRT measures the release of cytokines, histamine, leukotrienes, and prostaglandins released by white blood cells in response to inflammation. The theory behind MRT is that food sensitivity increases inflammation in the body, resulting in symptoms. Studies by the University of Miami, cited on the MRT website, report MRT testing is reliable. The ALCAT claims to measure food and other reactions to white blood cell production instead of antibodies. Because the reaction occurs at the cellular level, this test is thought to be more accurate. Results are controversial because IgG antibodies, which are created to fight certain allergenic foods, are also created in response to infections. Because they can be found in people who do not have allergies, it is speculated that they are a normal response to eating food. At this time reviews by the American Academy of Allergy, Asthma, and Immunology and the Food Allergy Research & Education organizations consider the MRT and ALCAT methods to be investigational. Both organizations recommend that more research into their accuracy is needed because of numerous subjective reports of accurate results in medical and nutritional practices.

Hair testing is another alternative allergy diagnosis method that has not shown promise when it comes to accuracy of results. A hair sample is taken from patients and tested for mineral content. The rationale of the test suggests that food allergies or sensitivities will alter the mineral content of their hair. However, hair grows very slowly, usually less than a half inch per month. Because of this, hair is not a good measure of mineral content, and this method of diagnosis is not recommended.

Pulse testing involves testing the pulse of patients after they eat a specific food. The pulse rate measures how fast the heart is beating. It was theorized by Dr. Arthur Coca that an allergic reaction to a food will increase heart rate and thus the pulse rate. There are no studies that validate this theory, and it is considered an unreliable test because there are many other factors that affect pulse rate, such as anxiety. Allergists do not recommend this test because of its unreliability.

8. How are food intolerances diagnosed?

Symptoms of food intolerances are often similar to those of food allergy, making diagnosis difficult. Except for a few food intolerances, there are currently no reliable test methods that diagnose them. Elimination diets are the only reliable testing method used currently to determine if an individual has a food intolerance. An elimination diet removes suspected foods from the daily diet for a two- to four-week period of time. If symptoms resolve, then it is concluded that there is an intolerance to that specific food. But the trigger food will usually be reintroduced into the diet, one at a time if there is more than one suspected food, to confirm the diagnosis. If symptoms reoccur, then an intolerance to that food or foods is confirmed. Reliable testing methods are available for fructose, lactose, sucrose, and sorbitol intolerances. The hydrogen breath test, lactose tolerance blood test, and stool acidity level are all used to diagnose a lactose intolerance. The hydrogen breath test is also used to confirm fructose, sucrose, and sorbitol intolerances.

The hydrogen breath test measures the amount of hydrogen found in the breath of the individual being tested. Normally there is little or no hydrogen present in the breath. But anaerobic bacteria that live in the colon will produce large amounts of hydrogen and methane when exposed to undigested food in the intestinal tract. These two excess gases will then be detected in the breath because the body removes them from the intestine into the bloodstream, which then eliminates it through the lungs. Prior to this test, an individual must fast (eat no foods or drinks except water) for at least 12 hours. An initial measurement of the breath is taken as a baseline measurement. Then the individual will drink a prepared lactose solution. Breath levels of hydrogen and methane will then be measured every 15 minutes from two to five hours after the lactose solution is taken. The amount of hydrogen and methane measured can then be used to confirm an intolerance. While the test is thought to be accurate, it diagnoses only an estimated 60 percent of food intolerances.

The lactose tolerance blood test measures how much sugar is in the blood two hours after drinking a lactose solution. The patient must fast (no food or drinks) for eight hours prior to the test. If blood glucose levels rise less than 20 mg/dl after two hours, the test is considered positive for lactose intolerance. For infants and young children, a stool acidity test will be used because of the difficulty of giving hydrogen breath or lactose tolerance blood tests to babies and young children. Undigested lactose forms lactic acid, which is measurable in a stool sample. Lactic acid detected in the stool confirms a lactose intolerance. It is important to note that antibiotics should not be taken for at least 30 days prior to testing because antibiotics decrease the amount of normal bacteria present in the large intestine, affecting the accuracy of test results. Small intestinal bacterial overgrowth, which is an abnormal amount of bacteria in the small intestine that is normally found in the colon, should also be ruled out prior to testing since it also produces lactose intolerance symptoms that usually resolve after treatment.

9. How are food sensitivities diagnosed?

Unlike food allergies and some food intolerances, traditional blood tests and small intestinal biopsies are usually negative for food sensitivities. Measuring blood levels of immunoglobulin G4 (IgG4), a measure of histamine levels and observed to increase when the immune system is exposed to food, has been used by some practitioners to diagnosis food sensitivities. However, increased IgG levels can be measured even without corresponding symptoms and are also seen when there is an infection. IgG4 is thought to identify exposure to a food but not necessarily tolerance to it. The European Academy of Allergy and Clinical Immunology concluded in 2008 that IgG4 testing for food sensitivities is not a reliable diagnostic test.

Lymphocyte response assay (LRA) by ELISA/ACT Biotechnologies is another test that some practitioners use to diagnose food sensitivities. This test should not be confused with the ELISA test, which is a valid and accurate test for certain infectious diseases. The LRA test appears to be based on the theory that food sensitivities are a Type IV hypersensitivity reaction. The LRA test mixes a patient's blood with more than 400 foods, minerals, preservatives, and other environmental substances. Lymphocyte levels are then measured in response to each substance. Elevated levels are concluded to confirm a food sensitivity. However, research has not validated the accuracy of the LRA test. Although it can measure some immune responses, elevations are not always caused by an immune system reaction, and therefore, the LRA is considered unreliable.

There are two other testing methods that some health-care practitioners use to diagnose food sensitivities. These are the Mediator Release Test (MRT) and the antigen leukocyte cellular antibody test (ALCAT). Both of these tests show promise in diagnosing food sensitivities but remain controversial as to accuracy. The MRT test evaluates 150 different foods and food additives. It measures the release of cytokines, histamine, leukotrienes, and prostaglandins, which are mast cell mediators released by white blood cells in response to inflammation and allergic reactions. A patient's blood is mixed with these foods and food additives in a test tube in the lab, and cell mediator levels are measured. Elevated levels indicate a food sensitivity. The theory behind MRT tests is that food sensitivity increases inflammation in the body and provokes the immune system to fight back, causing symptoms. Studies have yet to verify the MRT or ALCAT tests, however.

The Lifestyle, Eating, and Performance (LEAP) diet is frequently combined with MRT testing to confirm a suspected food sensitivity. LEAP is tailored specifically to the individual. Once MRT results are reviewed and specific foods are identified as possible sensitivities, the diet is planned for the patient, which eliminates each suspected food over a period of time. For example, MRT results are segregated and color coded into highly reactive (red), moderately reactive (yellow), and nonreactive (green) categories. During Phase I of the LEAP diet, the lowest nonreactive "green" foods are the only foods consumed for one week. During week 2, if there are no symptoms, Phase II begins by adding in the remaining green, yellow, and red foods one food at a time. A patient will remain in the Phase II period of the diet until all MRT reactive foods are added back into the diet. If all is going well, Phase III will add in other foods not tested on the MRT. Careful attention will be paid to symptoms, and any foods that do elicit a response will be assessed as a food sensitivity for that person. The LEAP diet also remains controversial and is not yet verified as an accurate diagnostic tool.

The ALCAT test, developed by Cell Science Systems, claims to measure food reactions to white blood cell production instead of antibodies. Leucocytes, which are white blood cells, are separated from a sample of a patient's blood and then added to 200 test food extracts. Reactivity to a specific food is determined by the leucocyte cell count for each food tested. Because the reaction occurs at the cellular level, this test is thought to be more accurate than the MRT test. A 2017 double-blind, randomized clinical trial of 58 patients with irritable bowel syndrome (IBS) at Yale

School of Medicine reported in the *BMJ Open Gastroenterology Journal* that patients following a specific elimination diet based on the results of a leucocyte activation test showed meaningful clinical improvement in symptoms of IBS. Study limitations included a small number of patients tested, homogenous population studied, and partial funding by Cell Science Systems.

To date, the American Academy of Allergy, Asthma, and Immunology considers both the MRT and ALCAT methods to be investigational, and research into their accuracy is still needed. The only reliable method of diagnosis for food sensitivities to date is the use of the elimination diet, as outlined previously.

10. What causes food allergies?

It is still unclear exactly why food allergies occur. A number of different theories about why someone does develop a food allergy have been proposed. Most of allergy research to date has been concentrated on the broken-skin hypothesis, the ingestion hypothesis, the helminth hypothesis, the hygiene hypothesis, the expanded hygiene hypothesis, and the toxin hypothesis.

The broken-skin hypothesis was formulated in 2003 after one study found exposure to low doses of peanut proteins introduced through broken or inflamed skin caused an allergic sensitization to peanuts. The Avon Longitudinal Study of Parents and Children at the University of Bristol in the United Kingdom found that refined peanut oil rubbed onto a child's skin that was open or inflamed subsequently caused an allergic reaction after eating peanuts, even though there was no evidence of peanut allergy at birth. The study concluded that sensitization to peanut could occur through exposure to small amounts of peanut through the skin. Follow-up studies in 2005, however, found that an equal number of children with eczema experienced peanut allergy reactions when compared with children who did not, failing to confirm this theory.

While the broken-skin hypothesis continues to be studied, this study did bring up a question about the use of refined peanut oils and other cross-reactive legume oils (e.g., castor oil and soybean oil) often used in oral and injected pharmaceuticals. Cross-reactivity reactions occur when an antibody directed at one protein is able to bind with another protein in another food because of their similar chemical structures. Unrefined peanut oil was used for decades in ointments for eczema and other skin conditions without a subsequent increase in peanut allergy cases. Vegetable oils were first refined during the mid-1900s to remove potentially harmful impurities. Processing of oils was crucial for safety as the proteins were well known to be allergenic and toxic. By 1913, emulsions of oils were stabilized with either egg lecithin or milk protein. This stabilized the mixture, making it less prone to break down and increased the amount of time it could be stored for use. As oil emulsions evolved, the product Lipomul was introduced in 1935 and was made with cottonseed oil. Cottonseed oils were increasingly used in processed foods and pharmaceuticals. Penicillin, the wonder drug of 1928 used to treat infections, was mixed with refined cottonseed oil for both injection and oral pills (a gelatin capsule) by 1944. Cottonseed oil slowed the excretion of penicillin by the kidneys, which was rapid without it. If given as a pill, it allowed the penicillin to bypass digestive enzymes, allowing delivery into the small intestine. Both outcomes improved the effectiveness of penicillin. But a sharp increase in cottonseed allergy reactions began to occur during the 1940s. In the 1950s the use of cottonseed oil in medicine and vaccines was eliminated, and a corresponding decrease in allergy reactions occurred. Cottonseed oil was replaced with a mixture of refined peanut oil and beeswax (POB) after World War II, and reported allergic reactions began to increase. In 1948 this mixture was replaced with a refined peanut oil and aluminum monostearate solution (PAM) that was in use throughout the 1980s. However, allergic reactions to PAM were significantly higher and more severe than those reported for PAM.

Refined peanut oil was approved for use in the United States in 1958 and considered a GRAS (generally recognized as safe) ingredient. GRAS food ingredients are food ingredients that the U.S. Food and Drug Administration has concluded to be safe for human consumption. Refined peanut oil was also used in many processed foods, medications, vitamins, skin creams, and infant formulas. The first study of peanut allergy in the United States occurred in 1973 when peanut allergy was noted to be a growing concern among children. However, it is important to note that peanut oil was used frequently in food, medicine, and fuel during the Civil War, both world wars, and the Depression because it was inexpensive and could be stored for long periods of time. During this same time period, no increase in the incidence of peanut allergies was seen. George Washington Carver (1864–1943), a prominent scientist and chemist, also used peanut oil as a massage therapy for polio patients for decades without a concurrent rise of peanut allergies during that time span. Although it appears there may be a connection between the use of refined peanut oil and allergy reactions, researchers have been unable to link the two, and there is still no clear answer if refined or unrefined oils used in everyday medications, vaccines, cosmetics, lotions, and other products are responsible for the increase in peanut sensitization.

To complicate this picture, use of highly refined oils is exempted from food labeling laws and not listed on food labels as potential allergens because they are generally regarded as safe. However, there have been reported incidences of children having an allergic reaction after taking an oral vitamin supplement or eating a baby formula that uses refined peanut oil in its formulation. Another theory about food allergies related to the use of highly refined oils proposes that some children become sensitized at birth from common injections that contain refined peanut, castor, or soybean oils. For example, in all Westernized countries, every newborn infant is given a vitamin K1 injection at birth. Vitamin K is an important vitamin that helps blood to clot, preventing serious bleeding incidents. While these incidents are rare, some infants have a rare bleeding disorder known as vitamin K deficiency bleeding (VKDB), which can cause brain damage or death. Newborns do not get enough vitamin K from their mothers prior to birth and do not start manufacturing sufficient amounts of Vitamin K on their own until they are approximately six months of age. The vitamin K shot is given as a preventive measure against VKDB. The vitamin K injection also contains refined peanut oil, having the potential to significantly increase sensitization to peanuts because of the large numbers of babies who receive these injections. However, no studies have been done to date to investigate this possible route of peanut sensitization. The FDA does report on its website that levels of peanut protein in refined peanut oils vary due to refining process differences. However, the FDA maintains that these differences are not of concern for public safety.

The ingestion hypothesis is another popular theory that posits that the time of life when peanuts are introduced into the diet may result in peanut sensitization if a child has a compromised digestive system or genes that cause a dysfunction of the Th1/Th2 immune response. It is well established that anaphylactic reactions were common among children given vaccines in the early 1900s. Dr. Charles Richet (1850–1935), a French immunologist, discovered what he termed "anaphylaxis." Allergic reactions to foods were uncommon at that time, but in the course of his research, Dr. Richet also discovered that food sensitization occurred when undigested proteins entered into the bloodstream. It was subsequently assumed that children who experienced anaphylaxis after eating a food had unhealthy digestive systems. Dr. Clemens von Pirquet's (1874–1929), a doctor at the Children's Clinic in Vienna, also suspected that undigested proteins injected into the bloodstream caused anaphylactic reactions.

Research efforts have identified the ability of proteins to increase IgE antibodies. Proteins are made of a strand of amino acids called epitopes. A medium-sized epitope of about 33 amino acids is required for an IgE antibody to connect with a mast cell. If a protein is smaller than this, it cannot connect with a mast cell and an allergy reaction cannot occur. Peanut proteins, identified as Ara h 1 and Ara h 2, and soybean proteins, identified as Gly m 1, have many allergenic epitopes that are capable of connecting with mast cells efficiently. Peanut proteins are also difficult to digest, increasing the risk of their passing into the bloodstream undigested and thus increasing risk for an allergic reaction. Boiling or frying peanuts appears to decrease the amount of Ara h 1 in peanuts versus dry roasting methods, which heat peanuts to high temperatures. Method of cooking peanuts appears to impact allergy reactions. This may account for the fact that peanut allergy is rarely seen in China, where peanuts are boiled, when compared to Westernized countries, where peanuts are roasted. However, the fact that peanuts have been eaten for years without an increase in peanut allergy until the time period between 1988 and 1994 (and worsening during the 2000s) in the United Kingdom, United States, Canada, and Australia indicates that something in the environment of children changed during this time frame to trigger a dramatic increase in peanut allergy cases.

The Th1/Th2 paradigm of the ingestion hypothesis involves the T cells of the immune system. There are two types of T cells, Type 1 and Type 2. Th1 cells make interleukin-2 (IL-2) and interferon. IL-2 and interferon are cytokines, which are proteins that regulate leukocyte activation against intracellular (inside the cell) bacteria, viruses, and parasites and disrupt their ability to replicate and spread. Th2 cells activate the immune system against intestinal helminthes (parasitic worms) and extracellular (outside the cell) parasites. Th1/Th2 cells produced by the immune system are considered the foundation of the immune response. When the Th1/Th2 paradigm is disrupted with high levels of Th1 and Th2 cells produced, the risk for autoimmune diseases and asthma increases. Subsequently, allergy reactions may possibly be correlated to this disruption.

The helminth hypothesis theorizes that helminthes, which are parasitic worms that live in the human body, coevolved with humans to protect humans from immune-mediated diseases, such as arthritis, inflammatory bowel disease, multiple sclerosis, and allergies. This theory was postulated after Neil Lynch discovered during the 1980s that 90 percent of Venezuelan Indians who lived in the rainforest had worm infections but no allergies. However, of the 10 percent of rich Venezuelans in the cities who had light worm infections, 43 percent had allergies. Helminthes are classified as roundworms (hookworms, *Trichinella*, eye worms) and flatworms (tapeworm, fluke). They burrow into the intestinal wall of their host and lay eggs. If infestation is excessive, they will spread into other areas of the body. It is suggested by researchers that helminthes suppress the immune system, making other proteins easy targets for IgE antibodies. However, other research findings indicate that while certain helminth infections can reduce allergy severity, they do not appear to prevent IgE antibody production to some allergens. In addition, children with heavy helminth infections can suddenly die from the toxins helminthes produce. Another flaw in this hypothesis is seen when it is realized that there are millions of people without helminth infestations who do not have IgE-mediated diseases. In general, helminth infections left untreated decrease the quality of life and shorten life spans of those who are infected. This hypothesis also does not explain the drastic increase in peanut allergies in Westernized countries since most individuals in Westernized countries do not experience helminth infections.

One environmental factor thought to be a significant cause of allergies is known as the hygiene hypothesis. The hygiene hypothesis proposes that Western and developing societies are "too clean." The human immune system is designed to fight infections, parasites, and harmful gut microorganisms. However, as Western and developing countries have evolved and improved hygiene and sanitation, individuals rarely have parasitic infections. Therefore, the immune system is idle and assumed to be "looking" for something to fight. It is thought the immune system begins to attack harmless proteins in food and air, resulting in allergy symptoms. This theory is supported by the fact that children who attend day care centers have lower asthma diagnosis rates when compared to children who do not attend them. Children born later in the birth order, have pets, or grow up on farms are also less likely to be diagnosed with allergies.

Dr. David Strachan proposed the hygiene hypothesis in 1989. Noting that family size was declining during the 1960s, Dr. Strachan found a correlation between an increased allergy prevalence and decreased exposure of germs of young siblings by older siblings. Increased exposure to germs by family members, friends, adults, and pets is theorized to strengthen the immune system. Dr. Strachan found the first birth in a family had a higher incidence of heightened immune response to common allergens than subsequent siblings in the birth order. His theory was further supported in 1989 when the Berlin Wall came down. East Germans were less strict about their hygiene habits and had lower vaccination rates, smoked tobacco, and were exposed to higher levels of pollution in their environment. However, they had lower allergy and asthma rates. But within a 10-year period of reuniting with West Germany, their allergy rates increased to the same levels of West Germans. It was extrapolated from this that absence of infections "reset" the immune system, which in turn caused abnormal reactions to foods and thus allergy development. Even so, the hygiene hypothesis fails to explain the drastic increase in peanut allergies since the 1990s. Evolutionary biologist Jared Diamond (1937) suggested many diseases were due to the fact that Europeans and other farming societies became infected with viral and bacterial pathogens due to their close proximity and handling of farm animals. This, in turn, led to the development of drugs, vaccines, and antibiotics to treat these diseases, leading in turn to immune imbalances that increase human susceptibility and allergic reactions.

The expanded hygiene hypothesis explores the destructive consequences of antibiotics on gut health and intestinal function. In 2014, the University of Chicago Medical Center studied the effect of clostridia, a common gut bacteria that exerts a reduction in sensitivity for allergies. This study treated mice with antibiotics that destroyed clostridia and then fed them peanuts. Blood samples from the mice showed an increase in IgE antibodies, indicating an allergic reaction to peanuts. After the mice were given clostridia to repopulate their gut, IgE antibodies specific to peanuts were reduced. The study authors found that "clostridia caused innate immune cells to produce high levels of interleukin-22 (IL-22), a signaling molecule known to decrease the permeability of the intestinal lining" ("Gut Bacteria That Protect against Food Allergies Identified," *Science Daily*, August 25, 2014). However, it is important to note that although the mice were sensitized to peanut, none of them experienced an allergic reaction after eating peanuts.

Another study compared children who had food allergies and those who did not between 2007 and 2009. Findings identified that children who were given a greater number of antibiotics had a higher risk for food allergies. Between 1988 and 1994, a time period when children had a significant increase in ear infections, high numbers of antibiotic prescriptions were given to children. While it is still unknown why this increase in ear infections occurred, many doctors and naturopathic practitioners attributed them to food allergies. A 1994 study published in the *Annals of Allergy* discovered that 86 percent of children had a significant reduction in ear infections when allergenic foods were eliminated from their diet. Ear, nose, and throat doctors have known for sometime that there is an association between a dairy allergy and ear infections. However, it is still unknown if the infection and antibiotics used to treat it caused the allergy or if the allergy caused the infection.

The toxin hypothesis proposed in 1991 by biologist Margie Profet theorizes that the human immune system has evolved to protect itself against acute toxicity and an allergy reaction is a protective mechanism against toxins. Toxins are found universally throughout the world, and humans have developed various ways to eliminate them. This includes remembering the smell to avoid them, eating a variety of fruits and vegetables to support elimination of them, and the body's removal of them via exhalation, feces, sweat, and urine. Dr. Profet theorizes that when the body is unable to remove specific toxins from the bloodstream, allergic reactions develop as a method to expel the toxins as quickly as possible. These allergic reactions include bronchial constriction, coughing, diarrhea, itching, sneezing, tearing, and vomiting. Peanuts are often contaminated with aflatoxin, which is a toxin produced from fungi and mold spores and often found on agricultural crops. Aflatoxins can be fatal and are considered a carcinogen. Dr. Profet theorizes peanut allergy reactions may actually be primarily associated with an IgE response to the aflatoxin and secondarily to the peanut protein associated with it. An allergy can be created when the body binds a toxin or carrier of a toxin with a serum protein. A 2007 study reported in *The Journal of Immunology* found mice were made allergic to peanuts when they inhaled or ate peanuts mixed with a bacterium. However, Dr. Profet states in her paper "The Function of Allergy" that food allergy is a complex process, and when two foods are consumed together the body may link them together in the digestive tract to elicit a toxic or immune response. Thus, years of exposure to hidden toxins in food such as additives or chemicals in beauty products, soaps, skin creams, antibacterial soaps, vaccines, and drugs may overwhelm the immune system and may make individuals more susceptible to allergies.

Other theories posit food protein shape, size, or folding pattern may trick the body into thinking it is an antigen. It is known that blood serum proteins must bond with a hapten, which is a molecule that elicits an immune response, to continue to circulate in the bloodstream (the kidneys are unable to filter them out), allowing the immune system to form antibodies to it. This theory speculates that a protein component found in the food-causing symptoms may have a unique shape, size, or folding pattern that fools the body into thinking it is an invader.

Another theory suspects that infants with food allergies may have an immature immune system, which doesn't allow them to distinguish between food proteins and harmful proteins in bacteria and viruses. It has been theorized that children born via caesarean section (C-section) may have a weaker immune system with a subsequent increased susceptibility for infections and allergies. During vaginal births the mother transfers essential bacteria to her newborn baby that strengthens the baby's immune system. Babies born by C-section do not receive this essential bacterial transfer, which may weaken their immune system making them more vulnerable.

Numerous studies find that inherited genes strongly influence whether a person develops a food allergy or not. Studies show a sevenfold increase in risk for developing a peanut allergy if an individual has a parent or sibling with peanut allergies. A small study of twins in 2000 by Scott H. Sicherer found 64 percent of identical twins developed peanut allergies in comparison to only 7 percent of nonidentical twins. Peanut allergies are estimated to have an 82 percent heritability factor. Food allergies are also strongly linked with allergy symptoms of asthma and atopic dermatitis. Asthma is a chronic disease of the lungs, causing difficulty breathing. Atopic dermatitis, also called eczema, is an inflammation of the skin that causes red, dry, itchy patches of skin. Studies suggest that genetic factors have a strong influence on the development of allergies other than foods, which manifest with these same symptoms. It is known that if both parents or one parent and one child in a family have significant allergies, then subsequent family members born into this family have an approximate 70–80 percent increased chance for developing an allergy. If only one parent has allergies, the allergy risk is reduced to about 40–50 percent. If a child has a sibling with an allergy, then the child has an estimated 15 percent increased risk for developing an allergy. Studies also find that if a child has an eczema triggered by an allergy that is moderate or severe, then he or she has an estimated 35 percent increased risk for developing a food allergy.

In 2001, the Human Genome Project announced the successful mapping of 90 percent of the genome sequence of the 3 billion base-pairs found in the human genome. This information was published in the journal *Nature* in February 2001. This has only been the beginning of understanding how genes influence human health and what treatments may manage them. To date genes associated with allergies include the *HLA-DRB1*, *HLA-DQB1*, *HLA-DPB1*, *CD14*, *FOXP3*, *STAT6*, *SPINK5*, *Interleukin 10*, and *Interleukin 13*. A December 5, 2017 study in the publication *Nature Communications* ("Integrative Transciptomic Analysis Reveals Key Drivers of Acute Peanut Allergic Reactions") identified six genes that turn on other genes in children with severe allergic reactions to peanuts. This study used a double-blind, placebo-controlled study (DBPC), which is considered the "gold standard" for research studies because it provides the strongest possible evidence for cause. In a DBPC study, subjects are assigned at random to a control group (those without an intervention) and an exposure group (those who are exposed to the study topic). Results are compared between the two groups. The December 5 gene DBPC study was the first study to identify specific genes responsible for peanut allergy reactions. This finding provides the possibility for targeted therapies that may be effective in the future. It is still important to remember that gene research is still in its infancy and much more research is needed to learn the significance of these connections and how best to manage them.

However, children in the same family and with the same genes do not always develop allergies. Because the incidence of food allergy has doubled over the past two decades and genes are unable to change that quickly, environmental factors also appear to play a role. The science of epigenetics researches changes that occur to inherited genes from the environment. These changes occur naturally all through the lifecycle but do not change the underlying DNA structure of the gene. Gene combinations act like recipes, which cells read and follow to function properly. Known as heritable changes, gene expression (the recipe) can be affected by environment, lifestyle, and the foods we eat. These environmental factors can cause an error in the gene "recipe," leading to chronic diseases or immune system malfunctions.

Other possible causes of food allergy that have been researched include the mother's diet during pregnancy, timing and introduction of solid foods to infants, and length of time infants are breastfed. Very few studies have been done exploring these areas, and those that have been done do not implicate the mother's diet during pregnancy or early feeding of infants as significant risk factors. In high-risk families, however, it does appear that breastfeeding for at least four to six months may reduce the development of allergies. More research is still needed in these areas, however.

The Institute of Medicine (IOM) reported a more controversial connection between food allergies and vaccines in 2011. The U.S. Department of Health and Human Services tasked the IOM with a review of medical and scientific evidence on the adverse effects of vaccines on health. The IOM report found a connection between vaccine ingredients and the development of food allergies. This is of particular concern in light of the fact that the Centers for Disease Control and Prevention doubled the recommended childhood vaccine schedule starting in the 1980s. A noted increase in childhood food allergies has been documented since the 1990s.

Serum sickness was a common reaction to the first mass injections of antitoxin sera for scarlet fever, tetanus, and diphtheria. Serum sickness is an allergic reaction to serum antitoxins found in vaccine ingredients, and symptoms include rashes, joint pain, fever, lymph node swelling, decreased blood pressure, enlarged spleen, kidney failure, difficulty breathing, shock, and death. Dr. Clemens von Pirquet and Dr. Béla Schick (1877–1967) both studied serum sickness among children injected with antitoxin serum. Dr. von Pirquet found that the symptoms of serum sickness were similar to allergic reactions to strawberries, crabs, pollens, bees, and mosquitoes. Subsequent vaccinations produced an exaggerated response (Clemens von Pirquet, "On the Theory of Infectious Diseases," unpublished paper deposited with the Imperial Academy of Sciences in April 1903). Dr. von Pirquet concluded that vaccination had two outcomes, immunity and hypersensitivity. He defined hypersensitivity as an altered immune reaction, which he termed an "allergy."

In 1964, the pharmaceutical company Merck began to use a new vaccine ingredient known as Adjuvant 65-4, created to be a safer adjuvant. An adjuvant is an additive to a vaccine that stimulates the body to produce antibodies against the viral or bacterial antigen in the vaccine. An adjuvant surrounds the vaccine antigens so that when the vaccine is injected into the muscle, the oil is gradually metabolized providing a sustained slow release of the other ingredients over a period of time. Injection into the muscle must be done properly, or allergy sensitization occurs if the injection goes into the bloodstream. Adjuvant 64-7 produced higher levels of antibodies than previous adjuvants. Adjuvant 65-4 contained peanut oil, Arlacel A, aluminum stearate, and other ingredients. Solutions of peanut oil combined with beeswax and peanut oil combined with aluminum monostearate were known to cause peanut allergies. Adjuvant 64-4 was also known to increase peanut sensitization since peanut proteins could not be entirely removed. Using Adjuvant 65-4 in vaccines was controversial among the medical community. It is currently assumed that Adjuvant 65-4 is not used in vaccines in the United States; however, it is unclear if this adjuvant is in use or not. Unfortunately, vaccinations have become a political issue, seriously impeding independent and unbiased investigation. What is clear is that vaccines have the potential to significantly alter the immune system and create hypersensitivity reactions that can cause an increased risk for other allergic reactions.

Transplants may also affect allergy status. One reported case in 2005 involved a child who underwent a bone marrow transplant for severe combined immune deficiency (SCID). SCID is a potentially fatal absence of functioning T and B lymphocytes of the immune system. Prior to the transplant the child had a peanut allergy. However, two years after the transplant, a food challenge showed the child to be peanut allergy free. While the exact mechanism for why this occurred is still not clear, it does indicate that the basic function of the immune system in this patient was changed by the transplant.

11. What causes food intolerances?

Food intolerances do not usually activate the immune system and mostly affect the gastrointestinal system. The inability to produce digestive enzymes that are necessary to break down foods into usable nutrients is the most common cause of food intolerances. However, aging; genetics; naturally occurring substances in food, chemicals, food additives; and food poisoning have also been implicated as reasons for food intolerance symptoms.

Normal digestion requires enzymes. Enzymes are protein molecules that induce and control the rate of specific chemical reactions in the body. There are two classes of enzymes, digestive and metabolic. Metabolic enzymes support and regulate biochemical reactions, generate energy, and repair organ and cell tissues. Digestive enzymes are essential for digesting foods properly and are secreted along the entire gastrointestinal tract, breaking down foods into a form that is readily absorbed and used by the body. Each enzyme has a specific function and type of food it breaks down. Amylase, lipase, proteases, and peptidases are the most common digestive enzymes the body produces to break down food. Amylase breaks down starchy foods, proteases and peptidases break down proteins, and lipases break down fats.

As people age, enzyme production in the body tends to decrease. Enzyme production may also decrease due to chronic health conditions. In some people genetics may prevent enzyme production. The result is improper digestion of foods, which causes food intolerance symptoms. The most common food intolerance is lactose intolerance. The National Digestive Diseases Information Clearinghouse estimates 30–50 million Americans are lactose intolerant. If lactase enzyme, a specific enzyme that breaks down lactose sugar found in milk or milk-based foods, is not present or there is a suboptimal amount of it in the digestive tract, lactose remains undigested and accumulates in the gastrointestinal tract. It then begins to be fermented by gut bacteria, which produces intolerance symptoms. There are three types of lactose intolerance: primary, secondary, and congenital. An individual is diagnosed with primary lactose intolerance if he or she does not have an underlying intestinal disease but develops intolerance symptoms due to a decreased amount of lactose available in his or her intestinal tract. Secondary lactose intolerance is caused by severe gastroenteritis, which is usually due to a virus that damages the intestinal mucosa temporarily. These cases often resolve after the person is well again and the intestine heals. Congenital lactose intolerance, such as galactosemia, is rare and due to a lifelong absence of the lactase enzyme because of a genetic defect. Galactosemia is a genetic disorder that affects the ability to process the simple sugar galactose, which is part of the larger lactose sugar molecule that is found in milk and dairy foods.

Besides lactase, there are many other specialty enzymes produced by the body to digest specific foods, and intolerances to any food can occur as a result. However, one interesting food intolerance is fructan intolerance. A 2018 Norwegian study published in the journal *Gastroenterology* found that fructans, which are short-chain carbohydrates, can cause gastrointestinal symptoms in susceptible individuals. Fructans are also called FODMAPs (fermentable oligosaccharides, disaccharides, monosaccharides, and polyols). These foods are carbohydrates, and if left undigested, they are fermented by intestinal gut bacteria producing gases that in turn produce symptoms. Oligosaccharides are found in wheat, rye, onion, garlic, and legumes. Disaccharides are lactose and found in milk and milk-based foods. Monosaccharides are fructose and found in honey, apples, and high-fructose corn syrup. Polyols are sorbitol and mannitol, found in some fruits and vegetables and also used in artificial sweeteners. What is of particular interest in this study is that many of these individuals are thought to be non-celiac gluten sensitive. Because fructans are found in wheat and rye, this study found that the individuals thought to be gluten sensitive were actually intolerant to fructans rather than gluten.

But food intolerances do not always involve digestive enzymes. Fructose is one example. In most people fructose is absorbed when it passes through the small intestine directly into the bloodstream without any need for a digestive enzyme. However, fructose intolerance can be the result of an inability to absorb fructose properly or because of an inherited gene. There are two types of fructose intolerance: hereditary fructose intolerance (HFI) and fructose malabsorption. HFI occurs as a result of a deficiency of the enzyme aldolase B, which is produced by the liver. When fructose is absorbed directly through the small intestine wall, aldolase B turns it into glucose that the body uses immediately for energy. When a person does not inherit the ability to make aldolase B, fructose is absorbed into the bloodstream but does not undergo the change to glucose. Fructose then begins to collect in the liver and kidneys, causing severe hypoglycemia (low blood sugar). Hypoglycemia symptoms include anxiety, fatigue, heart palpitations, hunger, irritability, and shakiness. Fructose intolerance can also occur when fructose cannot be absorbed because it cannot pass through the small intestinal wall, resulting in an accumulation of it in the intestine. When fructose accumulates, gastrointestinal bacteria attempt to digest it through the process of fermentation, which then produces symptoms.

Sometimes added or naturally occurring chemicals in foods and drinks can prompt intolerance symptoms. One culprit is known as the "cheese effect" and is the result of amines. Amines form when protein foods are broken down during the digestive process. Amines are known to be vasoactive, which affects the diameter of blood vessels that then increases or decreases blood pressure or heart rate. Vasoactivity may also slow down or speed up the transit of foods through the intestine. Vasoactive amines are histamine, phenylethylamine, serotonin, tyramine, and tryptamine. They can be found naturally in some foods, such as anchovies, bananas, aged cheeses (e.g., blue cheese and Cheddar cheese), chocolate, smoked fish, cured meats, some beers, sausage, spinach, tomato, tuna, wine, yeast extracts, and fermented foods. They can also be produced during conventional cooking processes and during food storage. For instance, increased levels of tyramine, an amino acid found in protein foods, can be found in foods stored for long periods of time or that have not been refrigerated at the proper temperature. Foods highest in natural amounts of histamine and tyramine are fermented foods, alcohol, cheese, sauerkraut, sausage, and canned tuna.

Histamine, produced by the immune system when activated to destroy foreign microorganisms that could be dangerous, can also be found in foods that have not been stored properly. Improperly stored fish is one example. When fish becomes old and begins to go bad, histamine levels increase. Eating spoiled food may lead to intolerance symptoms and sometimes the deadly allergic reaction of anaphylaxis known as scombroid poisoning. Scombroid poisoning most commonly occurs in improperly refrigerated tuna or mackerel fishes. Histamine constricts blood vessels and the muscle of the intestine and lungs, increasing heart rate, lowering blood pressure, and causing symptoms of asthma, headache, and skin flushing and, if severe enough, anaphylaxis.

Besides protein foods, tyramine is found in prescription drugs that contain monoamine oxidase (MAO) inhibitors, such as some blood pressure and antidepressant medications. MAOs are the enzymes normally used to break down amines. Some individuals are born without the MAOA gene, and their gastrointestinal tract will not produce MAO. These individuals cannot break down amines, which results in a buildup of tyramine in the bloodstream. The buildup of tyramine in turn causes a narrowing of blood vessels, which can produce the release of histamine and prostaglandins to counteract it. This in turn produces symptoms that can sometimes be life threatening, such as chest pain, confusion, severe headache, high blood pressure, nausea, nosebleeds, shortness of breath, vision changes, and vomiting. It is also thought that tyramine may trigger migraines; however, studies have not conclusively confirmed this. Some individuals may also produce low amounts of MAO enzymes, known as MAOA-L, which has been observed to cause aggressive or violent behavioral symptoms. Those lacking the MAOA gene or producing too little of MAO will be advised to follow a low-tyramine diet.

One naturally occurring substance found in some foods is caffeine. Caffeine is found in coffee, tea, and chocolate. Caffeine-sensitive individuals may experience symptoms of intolerance when they ingest caffeine because of its pharmacological diuretic effect. A diuretic effect increases the rate of fluid removal from the body and relaxes blood vessels, which then lowers blood pressure.

Naturally occurring toxins in foods may also affect sensitive individuals and produce intolerance symptoms. For example, undercooked beans can cause digestive problems because they have a compound called aflatoxin, which ferments in the gastrointestinal tract if inadequately digested. Aflatoxins are chemicals produced by specific molds that grow in soil, decaying vegetation, hay, and grains. Aflatoxins are found naturally in peanuts, beans, lentils and other beans, pistachios, cereals that contain raw seeds and nuts, maize, some dried fruits and figs, black pepper, chilies, and spices. Foods considered to be a high risk for aflatoxins are extremely toxic and carcinogenic and may cause death. Most countries strictly regulate these foods. Legumes, such as peanuts, and other risky foods are inspected for mold, which are eliminated from the food supply or chemically decontaminated. Cooking beans properly, which does not completely eliminate aflatoxins, will usually break down the legume and reduce the toxic effect enough that an individual is able to digest it properly. Sensitive individuals are often able to eat fully cooked beans without symptoms.

Salicylate intolerance occurs when the immune system overreacts to normal amounts of salicylates found in foods. Salicylates are derivatives of salicylic acid. Salicylic acid occurs naturally in plants and is a plant's immune system, using salicylic acid to defend against bacteria, fungi, insects, and disease. Most fruits and vegetables, spices, herbs, flavor additives, and tea have naturally occurring salicylates, although some of these more processed foods may have them added. Mint flavors, tomato sauce, berries, processed foods, and citrus fruits have the highest levels of salicylates.

Sometimes food additives cause an individual to have symptoms of intolerance. Food additives have been used for centuries as a way to preserve foods. Salt, spices, and sugar were natural preservatives used along with fermentation and smoking of foods. But as countries became more Westernized and industrialization became a way of life with increasing numbers of people moving to cities to work in factories, food preservation techniques were needed. Food additives that preserved or colored foods were common by 1820. As of 1830, sodium nitrate was used to preserve butter and meats, and sulfites and acetates were used to preserve meats. Concerns about food additive safety led to the formation of the Poison Squad in the United States. The Poison Squad was a group of 12 men who volunteered to test the safety of food additives for the Agriculture Department (later renamed the Food and Drug Administration) in 1902. For five years these men ate nightly meals prepared by a government kitchen in which food preservatives were added. Each participant was observed, and weight, temperature, and pulse were recorded before every meal. Stool and urine samples were collected, and symptoms of sickness were recorded. The Poison Squad was disbanded in 1907 after it was determined that the food additives they had tested were harmful to their health.

In 1958 the United States passed regulations that required food and chemical manufacturers to test their food additives for safety. A generally recognized as safe (GRAS) list was formulated of those additives thought to be safe for human consumption. As of 1980, 415 different substances were approved as safe food additives. The use of food additives has increased dramatically since the 1950s as more and more foods are now processed and available on supermarket shelves. Food additives are used in processed foods to enhance food flavor, make foods look more appealing, and increase the shelf life of a food product. The use of food additives in our food supply appears to be impacting sensitive individuals more than in the past. The most common additives added to foods are antioxidants, artificial colors and flavorings, emulsifiers, flavor enhancers, preservatives, and sweeteners. Nitrate additives are found in processed meats and known to cause itching and skin rashes. Sodium nitrite is used as a food additive because it is an antibacterial agent. In large amounts, specified as 20 mg or more, it can dilate blood vessels and produce intolerance symptoms of skin flushing, headache, and urticaria. Monosodium glutamate is used as a flavor enhancer, often found in Chinese meals, and known to cause headaches. Sulfites are used as a food preserver or enhancer and found most often in wines. Sulfites are also known to trigger symptoms of intolerance in susceptible individuals. Food colorings, especially red (carmine) and yellow (annatto), are also known to produce intolerance symptoms in sensitive individuals.

12. What causes food sensitivities?

Food intolerances and food sensitivities are all interconnected and, in general, have many of the same symptoms, making diagnosis difficult. There are many theories about why they occur, but research is still ongoing in this area. Reactions to foods are either immediate and IgE mediated, as in a food allergy, or delayed and non-IgE mediated or IgG mediated. Type I hypersensitivity reactions are associated with severe reactions and food allergies. Type II hypersensitivity is usually IgG mediated but has not been associated with food reactions. Type III hypersensitivities affect either the body, in general, such as serum sickness, or specific individual organs. Type III reactions may occur 3–10 hours after antigen exposure, and at this time there does not appear to be a connection to food sensitivity reactions. Type IV hypersensitivity, however, appears to possibly be the root cause for many autoimmune diseases. Type IV symptoms usually occur 48–72 hours after antigen exposure, and this delayed reaction is thought to be tied to food sensitivities because of the length of time it takes for symptoms to appear.

The immune system has also been found to have gut-associated lymphoid tissue (GALT) in the intestine. The GALT system is found to be a backup defense against food antigens. The GALT system can decrease the permeability of the intestine and allows a tolerance or elimination of antigens passing through it. But the GALT system has also been found to promote intestinal damage in diseases such as celiac disease, inflammatory bowel disease, and food allergy.

Many specific and medically recognized autoimmune diseases or disorders have been connected to food sensitivity reactions. More controversial within the medical community is leaky gut syndrome. A leaky gut is also known as intestinal hyper-permeability or dysbiosis, and a number of theories have been suggested for why it occurs.

One common theory for leaky gut is hyper-permeability of intestinal junctions, which are gastrointestinal cells found along the walls (mucosa) of the small and large intestines. Intestinal junctions are normally very tightly connected, which keeps bacteria, toxins, microbes, and undigested food particles out of the bloodstream. But loose junctions appear to create "holes" in the intestinal tract that allow undigested or toxic substances to pass through. Because these substances would not normally be allowed to pass through into the bloodstream, they increase inflammation and irritation in body systems causing illnesses or sensitivity symptoms. In general, once intestinal junctions and leaky gut are healed, food sensitivities are often reported to resolve.

Another theory links leaky gut to dysbiosis, which is an imbalance of "good" bacteria to "bad" bacteria in the intestinal tract. Chronic gastrointestinal diseases or constant exposure to trigger foods can damage intestinal cells, causing a bacterial imbalance. Antibiotic medications may also destroy good bacteria, leaving behind an overabundance of bad bacteria that can negatively affect health. The result of this imbalance is an increase in systemic inflammation that causes symptoms.

It is now known that 70 percent of the entire immune system resides in the intestine. The GALT system comprises an estimated 80 percent of immunoglobulin cells.

Research is beginning to show that the gastrointestinal tract is considered to be our "second brain" and contributes much more to immunity than previously recognized. A 2017 research report in the journal *Frontiers in Immunology*, "Leaky Gut as a Danger Signal of Autoimmune Diseases," reported that cells underneath the intestinal lining contain B and T cells, along with other immune-related cells. The antibody IgA has also been found to reside primarily on the surface of the intestinal mucosa. Known as secretory IgA (SIgA), it is uniquely resilient to digestive enzymes. This resilience allows SIgA to effectively protect against pathogens. When infections affect the digestive tract, it appears that gastrointestinal symptoms may actually be caused by the immune response that occurs within the gastrointestinal tract. While symptoms of food sensitivities can be the same as allergy reactions, they are also thought to trigger chronic conditions such as asthma, autism, autoimmune diseases, eczema and psoriasis, inflammatory bowel disease, rheumatoid arthritis, systemic inflammatory response syndrome, and type I diabetes as well as joint pains or "brain fog."

A more controversial theory for food sensitivity reactions is the increased use of genetically modified foods (GMOs) in the modern-day food supply. GMOs are foods that are modified from their natural genetic structure. The genetic material of a plant, animal, bacteria, or virus is re-engineered in a lab, changing its genetic makeup. GMOs were first developed in plants during the 1980s, and the first FDA-approved GMO plants approved for commercial use in the United States occurred in 1994. GMOs were created to increase crop yields and strengthen a plant's resistance to bacteria, toxins, and insects. The resulting seed grew a hardier plant that produced more food and could survive insect infestations and drought conditions. The top GMO crops and foods in the United States as of 2018 include alfalfa, aspartame, corn, canola oil, cotton, milk, papaya, potatoes, soy, sugar beets, sugar, zucchini, and yellow squash. As of 2017, a GMO salmon and GMO apple were allowed on the market, and a GMO beef is expected to be available soon. GMO use in the U.S. food supply has increased dramatically since 1994. It is theorized that the gastrointestinal tract cannot recognize these genetically altered foods, leading to difficulty digesting them that in turn causes a food sensitivity reaction. The data about GMO safety is controversial, with some studies indicating GMO foods are not harmful to human health and other studies indicating they are harmful. The lack of impartial research about their safety is suboptimal, and unfortunately, GMOs are a political issue as well. More research is needed about their safety, but it is of interest to note that many European countries have banned GMO crops and foods for human consumption. Currently 38 countries have a ban on GMO foods and/or restrictions on imports that are GMO.

To date, no clear root cause for food sensitivities has been discovered for exactly why an individual becomes sensitive when others do not. Aging, chronic autoimmune diseases, environmental toxic overload, genetics, viral or bacterial infections, stress, or repeated exposures to a food or chemical are all thought to be possible triggers that damage the mucosa of the gastrointestinal tract. The typical American diet, which tends to be low in fiber and high in sugar and saturated fats, is also thought to impair the functioning of the intestinal tract.

13. Is there an environmental connection among the development of food allergies, intolerances, and sensitivities?

Genetic makeup appears to strongly influence whether an individual develops food reactions or not. However, genes do not change quickly from generation to generation. Genes are made of deoxyribonucleic acid (DNA), which is a set of instructions that cells read and follow to function properly. DNA is shaped like a ladder whose structure is made of molecules, called bases, known as adenine (A), thymine (T), guanine (G), and cytosine (C). Every person inherits two copies of this DNA "alphabet," one from each parent. Approximately 99 percent of genes are the same for everyone in the world. But slight variations in the remaining 1 percent of genes contain the small differences that give individuals their unique physical attributes that distinguish them from everyone else.

The A base always pairs up with the T base, and the G base always pairs up with the C base as a general rule. Because every cell in the body contains a complete set of DNA instructions, DNA is constantly being copied as new cells replace old ones. A single nucleotide polymorphism (SNP) is a copying error that can occur during this process, pairing bases differently from the rule. For instance, A may pair up with C instead of T as the result of a copying error. When the bases pair incorrectly, genetic susceptibility for diseases or other conditions is increased. But this does not mean an individual will definitely develop a disease. Other factors also affect genes or gene SNP combinations that can either "turn on" a susceptible gene, causing a chronic disease or immune system malfunction, or reduce the risk for a disease.

The science of epigenetics investigates the changes that can occur to inherited genes as a result of environmental influences. These changes occur naturally throughout the lifecycle without changing the underlying DNA structure of the gene. Research is finding that environmental factors can change the instructions in the cell, called a heritable change. Because the number of reported food allergies, intolerance, and sensitivity reactions has increased significantly over the past two decades, and genes are not able to change this quickly, environmental factors are strongly implicated in negative reactions to food. Numerous environmental theories have been explored.

Environmental exposure to peanuts during infancy is one theory surmised to increase the risk for peanut allergies. However, a 2015 research study reported that avoidance of peanuts in young babies and children actually increased the likelihood of developing a peanut allergy. Until this report it was recommended that families with a history of peanut allergy avoid all environmental exposures to peanuts and peanut products from infancy. The LEAP (Learning Early About Peanut) study demonstrated that infants at high risk for developing peanut allergies could actually prevent their peanut allergy by eating peanut-containing snacks as an infant. Because of the results of the LEAP study, healthcare practitioners are now recommending that peanuts should be introduced into the diet early in life. The U.S. Food and Drug Administration (FDA) approved the first food product that may help prevent peanut allergy. "Hello, Peanut" is a powder of organic peanuts and oats that can be mixed with pureed baby food and given to infants soon after they begin to eat solid foods, around the age of six months. Small amounts of the powder are started, gradually increased over a week, and then maintained until the child begins to eat peanut butter. However, allergy testing prior to introducing this product is strongly recommended if the infant has severe eczema or an egg allergy and should only be started with doctor supervision.

Environmental exposures that impair the gastrointestinal system have also been suspected to play a significant role in the development of allergies. Enzyme production throughout the gastrointestinal tract is essential to catabolize proteins properly so that intact proteins do not pass through the gut lining into the bloodstream. The passing of intact proteins through the gut into the blood can result in sensitization and an allergic reaction. Dr. Kenneth Bock suggested in his 2007 book, *Healing the New Childhood Epidemics, Autism, ADHD, Asthma and Allergies*, that a low-grade infection from environmental toxins, such as vaccinations, affects the gastrointestinal tract adversely, resulting in allergy sensitization. This in turn causes an infection that may send out immune cell messengers. These messengers then trigger inflammation in other parts of the body that contribute to allergy symptoms. It is known that patients with inflammatory bowel disease, such as celiac disease, show an IgE-mediated allergy to digestive microflora. Inflammation in the gastrointestinal tract may also inflame eosinophilic airways, frequently identified in those with peanut allergies. This occurs when eosinophils cross into the trachea and build up along the airways.

A more controversial environmental connection involves vaccinations. The U.S. Department of Health and Human Services tasked the Institute of Medicine (IOM) to review medical and scientific evidence on the adverse effects of vaccines on health. The IOM reported in 2011 that a connection between vaccine ingredients and the development of food allergies was found. This is of particular concern in light of the fact that the Centers for Disease Control and Prevention (CDC) doubled the recommended childhood vaccine schedule since the 1980s, with a noted increase in childhood food allergies in the 1990s.

Vaccine adjuvants have also been suspected of causing allergy reactions. An adjuvant is used in vaccines to make them more potent and effective at preventing illness. Because the majority of vaccines used today use only a small amount of weakened or dead pathogens as the antigen being vaccinating against, an adjuvant is also used to activate the immune system to work with the antigen to induce a long-term protective immunity. The immune system has innate immunity and adaptive immunity. Innate immunity occurs within a few hours of exposure to a pathogen. Adaptive immunity develops over several days with the activations of T and B cells. Adjuvants affect adaptive immunity, and antigens affect innate immunity. Aluminum salts or gels are the most widely used adjuvants in vaccines as well as peanut oil. It is known that no vaccine is 100 percent risk free and, while risk is thought to be low, it is also well known that the immune system of some individuals can become inflamed and hypersensitive. Adjuvants strongly activate immune receptors that have the potential to induce chronic immune activation and inflammation that does not stop post-immunization. This in turn can increase susceptibility to allergic reactions.

Cross-sensitization with other pollens has also been connected with food allergies. A 2008 Swedish study highlighted this connection. While peanuts are not a common food staple in Sweden, peanut allergy incidence is high. Swedish researchers suspected that individuals who had birch pollen allergies also had an increased risk for peanut allergies due to oral allergy syndrome. In 1959, research confirmed in mice that grass pollen, used as an adjuvant in pertussis vaccines, caused an immune response. A similar study in 1973 concluded that mice became sensitive to ragweed pollen after vaccination with a pertussis vaccine that caused an anaphylactic reaction. A subsequent study in 2005 was able to produce a peanut allergy in mice when peanut was mixed with a toxic bacterium that was inhaled via an adjuvant.

Some studies point to seasonal environmental reasons that may increase the risk for food allergy. One study discovered that 55 percent children born between the months of January and March had their first peanut allergy reaction during those same months. Fifty-seven percent of children born between October and December also experienced their first reactions during those same months. However, this did not occur in children born between April and June. It was speculated that diet changes on or near a child's first birthday could possibly have an impact. However, this theory has yet to be confirmed.

In 2000, researchers discovered that gender played a significant role for food allergy risk. Peanut allergy cases were found to be much higher for males than females by 2:1. A Duke University study that evaluated children born between 1988 and 1999 and 2000 and 2005 found 66 percent of those with peanut allergies were male. A subsequent Australian study found 60 percent of those with food allergy under the age of five were male. Only one 2008 study, by the CDC, found males and females were equally susceptible to food allergy. Research does find that overall males are more susceptible to environmental contaminants than females. A 2003 study confirmed this finding by evaluating a community in Ontario, Canada, that is downriver from petrochemical plants that released pollutants into the water supply. The birthrate of boys in this community was decreased in comparison with female births, which outnumbered male births by 2:1. The study concluded that these environmental pollutants had a negative impact on males. An increased risk for food allergy in males has also been seen in those with an increased risk for autism and Asperger's syndrome.

Children born by cesarean section (C-section) rather than vaginally are theorized to have an increased risk for food allergies. A child born by C-section is deprived of important bacterial microflora that is transferred via the vaginal canal during the birth process. The result is a bacterial imbalance in the gastrointestinal tract that impacts the immune system. Another theory posits the use of antibiotics to prevent infections after a C-section may alter intestinal bacteria. A Finland study found allergic children had different fecal bacteria when compared to children without allergies. Allergic children were most commonly deficient in lactobacillis and bifidobacteria microbial strains. Studies that prescribed children born by C-section prebiotics and probiotics over a five-year period experienced less Ig-E-associated immune sensitivities. While studies indicate that C-section birth appears to increase the risk for allergies, there are still no specific links between C-section birth methods and peanut allergies.

Another possible environmental influencer for allergies is the increased use of genetically modified foods in the food supply. One example of a possible connection between food allergy and GMOs occurred in the 1990s when genes from Brazil nuts were used to enhance soy beans. The Brazil nut gene was used to provide a genetically altered and improved protein in soy beans. However, a University of Nebraska study found that individuals allergic to Brazil nuts also had serious allergic reactions to the GMO-altered soy bean. While it seems to be common sense to expect that this could occur, regulation of GMOs in the United States actually increased the risk for a consumer to experience an allergy reaction. Currently food technology and manufacturing labeling is voluntary with regard to GMOs. Therefore, it is possible that a person eating a food that he or she considers to be safe may actually be exposed to an allergen without his or her knowledge. The other possible risk is the creation of a protein previously unknown that has unknown effects on humans. However, these theories still do not account for the rapid increase in peanut allergies.

Another concern regarding GMOs is the use of the chemical glyphosate. Commonly called Roundup, glyphosate is an herbicide used to destroy weeds growing up around crops without harming the actual plant being grown. Weeds crowd out the growing plant, resulting in the death of the plant or a decrease in crop yield. Roundup was first used in 1974 to alter a normal plant's ability to grow. GMO plants were approved for use in the United States in 1995 so these plants would be resistant to Roundup while also continuing to grow while the weeds around them were killed. Plants use the enzyme shikimate pathway, which is found only in microorganisms and plants, to make the essential amino acids phenylalanine, tyrosine, and tryptophan. These essential amino acids in the plant are crucial for growth. Because this pathway is not found in animals and humans, it was assumed glyphospate would not harm humans. However, it has since been discovered that glyphospate does interfere with bacteria in the human digestive tract because the common bacteria found in the intestine also use the shikimate pathway. Dr. Stephanie Seneoff of the Massachusetts Institute of Technology has found in her research that Roundup impairs the transport of sulfate and other enzymes needed for detoxification pathways in the human body. Detoxification pathways remove toxins from the body. It is theorized from this research that glyphospate impairs the health integrity of the microbiome, which can cause leaky gut and an increased risk for food sensitization with increased IgE levels.

Other popular environmental theories thought to cause food allergies and sensitivities and previously discussed include the broken-skin hypothesis, the hygiene hypothesis, the ingestion hypothesis, the helminth hypothesis, the expanded hygiene hypothesis, and the toxin hypothesis. But none of these theories has yet been confirmed as the root cause for adverse food reactions.

14. Are food allergies, sensitivities, and intolerances permanent?

Most food allergies are usually permanent if not outgrown by age five. However, there is clinical evidence that egg, milk, soy, and wheat allergies may still be outgrown by adulthood. Allergies to fish, peanuts, shellfish, and tree nuts are less likely to be outgrown. Children with multiple food allergies and severe immune reactions are also less likely to outgrow a food allergy. Food allergies that develop during adulthood are usually permanent.

Allergy researcher, Ruchi Gupta, found 41 percent of milk allergies, 40 percent of egg allergies, 16 percent of peanut allergies, and 13 percent of shellfish allergies were most likely to be outgrown by age 10. Children likely to outgrow tree nut allergies often did so by age 10 and shellfish allergies by age 12. Other researchers have confirmed Gupta's findings and also report 22 percent of peanut allergies are outgrown between the ages of 4 and 20. Sixty-five percent outgrow wheat allergies by the age of 12. Approximately 9 percent of children outgrow tree nut allergies by age five.

Peanut allergy is one of the most common food allergy reactions reported among children during the first few years of life. While it is usually a lifelong allergy, researchers Nasser Al-Ahmed et al. found that 15–22 percent of children outgrow their peanut allergy before their teenage years. They also found that in patients with a history of peanut allergy and peanut-specific IgE levels of five or less, they had a 50 percent chance of outgrowing their peanut allergy.

As a child becomes older, his or her allergist will monitor symptoms and accidental reactions, recommending testing and a medically supervised food challenge test if indicated. Younger children, whose immune system changes more rapidly than older children, are often tested every 6–12 months in comparison to older children. Testing includes skin tests and blood tests that measure food-specific IgE antibodies. If appropriate, the allergenic food may be fed to the child in small amounts under close medical supervision.

Food challenge tests are used very cautiously and infrequently because of the increased risk for a life-threatening anaphylactic reaction. However, a 2017 study in the *Annals of Allergy, Asthma, & Immunology* found that 86 percent of food challenges resulted in no adverse reactions and 98 percent of challenges had no symptoms of anaphylaxis. It is recommended that children with food allergies be periodically retested, especially if they were diagnosed at a young age.

Food sensitivities and intolerances may also resolve over time, especially after recovery from a viral or bacterial infection or illness. For some people, healing a "leaky gut" may eliminate the food sensitivity or intolerance permanently. However, if symptoms are the result of inflammatory bowel diseases, because of an enzyme deficiency, or due to an autoimmune disease, then sensitivities and intolerances will usually be lifelong. Those with FPIES or food protein-induced enterocolitis or proctocolitis often outgrow it within one to three years. Oral food allergies, sulfite-induced asthma, and food-dependent, exercise-induced anaphylaxis patients usually remain sensitive and must constantly be vigilant about their diet and the foods they eat.

15. Are certain groups of individuals more susceptible to negative food reactions?

Negative food reactions affect children and adults of all races and ethnicities. There are no hard-and-fast rules about who will or can develop a negative reaction to a food, but genetics and environment appear to have the most influence on increased susceptibility for them. It appears more likely that, even though race is not seen as a strong risk factor for food allergy, disparities in care and socioeconomic factors among the races may possibly skew what available data there is about this area of research. To date, very little data has been collected regarding ethnicity and food allergies.

In an effort to evaluate if there was a difference, the American Academy of Allergy Asthma & Immunology reported about a 2013 systematic review of available data conducted by researchers at the University of Michigan, the Centers for Disease Control and Prevention, the Food Allergy Research and Education Network, and the Massachusetts General Hospital. In this review, only black and white children in the United States were looked at, and the available data that was evaluated involved confirmed food allergy diagnosis cases, lab evidence confirming sensitization, caregiver-reported food allergies without clinical evidence, and medical care utilization that indicated possible food allergy reactions. Of 20 studies that were identified, 14 studies indicated a possible association between black children and a higher incidence of food allergy. However, most of these studies had design flaws and limitations that made results inconclusive. Overall the researchers concluded that it was not possible to accurately assess if black children are more susceptible than white children for developing a food allergy based on the existing available data.

The National Center for Health Statistics (NCHS) also evaluated trends in allergy cases in the United States from 1997 through 2011. It found that allergy reactions were the most common medical conditions affecting children in the United States. The most common allergies affecting children were food, skin, and respiratory allergies. All three categories reported an increase in allergies over this 14-year time span. In children between ages 0 and 17 years, food allergies increased from 3 percent in 1997 to 5 percent by 2011. Hispanic children were found to have a lower rate of food allergies (3.5%) compared to non-Hispanic whites (5%) and non-Hispanic black (a little over 5%) children. The differences in food allergy rates between non-Hispanic whites and non-Hispanic black children were statistically insignificant.

The NCHS also looked at income levels and allergy rates. It found that children in families with an income less than 100 percent of the poverty level were less likely to have food allergies when compared with families with higher incomes. Four percent of children living in families with an income less than 100 percent of the poverty level were reported to have food allergies. Five percent of children in families with an income 100–200 percent of poverty level were reported to have food allergies. Above

200 percent of poverty level, almost 5.5 percent of children were reported to have a food allergy. The NCHS concluded that the prevalence of food allergies did increase during this time span, with Hispanic children having the lowest food allergy rates, and that income levels appeared to influence the number of children who developed food allergies.

16. What is the prevalence of food allergies in the United States and in the world?

Food allergy prevalence is estimated by allergy and world health organizations because most of the available data about food allergy incidence is self-reported by individuals or their family members. Confirming skin or blood tests may or may not be done, and the diagnostic method of double-blind, placebo-controlled food provocation test is not routinely evaluated. According to the World Allergy Organization (WAO), as of 2013, an estimated 220–250 million people had a food allergy worldwide. Of these, 5–8 percent were estimated to be children and 1–2 percent adults. The main allergens that affect the majority of developed countries include egg, milk, peanut, fish and shellfish, soy, tree nuts, and wheat. But other allergens may be common in a specific country based on popular foods and dishes of that culture and how they are processed. For example, allergy to sesame seeds is much more common in Israel and Arab nations than in Westernized countries where peanut allergies are more common.

While sesame seeds are a staple of the Israeli and Arab diet in comparison to peanuts, which are a staple food in America, it is also possible that the way peanuts are prepared in each country makes a difference in allergy response. In America and most Westernized countries, peanuts are roasted. In Israel and Arab countries, peanuts are boiled. Peanuts have three major allergens, Ara h 1, Ara h 2, and Ara h 3. Those with peanut allergy in the United States are most commonly allergic to Ara h 2. The process of roasting peanuts is shown to increase IgE antibody reactions to Ara h 2. In comparison, boiling peanuts exposes the peanut to the heat process for longer periods of time, which is shown to decrease Ara h 2 levels. Peanuts are usually roasted in the United States, which may explain why Americans have a more common and more severe allergic reaction to peanuts than if they were boiled. This is one area where more research is needed, however.

According to the Food Allergy Research & Education Association, more than 170 different foods have been reported to cause an allergic reaction in the United States. From 1994 to 2006 the most common food allergens reported in the United States were to egg, milk, peanut, fish and shellfish, soy, tree nuts, and wheat. As of 2015, researchers estimated that up to 15 million Americans had at least one food allergy. Of these, almost 6 million were children under the age of 18, and approximately 30 percent of them had multiple food allergies. Few studies have examined the prevalence of food sensitivities and intolerances to date. It is unknown how many children and adults struggle with them.

In an attempt to gain more objective information Dr. Li Zhou, a lead researcher at Brigham and Women's Hospital, and her colleagues reviewed almost 3 million medical records involving patients treated for allergic reactions from 2000 to 2013. Their results were reported in the December 2017 *Journal of Allergy and Clinical Immunology*. Dr. Zhou and her colleagues identified more than 97,000 patients who experienced one or more food allergy or intolerance episodes over this 13-year time span. Females experienced more allergic reactions than males, and the most common food allergies were to shellfish, specific fruits and vegetables, dairy, and peanuts.

A review by the WAO in 2012 surveyed 89 countries in an attempt to identify global patterns of food allergy prevalence. Only half of the countries surveyed collected data regarding food allergy in their country. Nine of the 89 countries studied kept accurate food allergy prevalence data that was also confirmed by oral food challenges. Twenty-three of the 89 countries collected data that was based on parent-reported symptoms, which is universally recognized as overestimating food allergy cases. In total, data was collected from 12 Western European countries, 5 Nordic countries, 17 Central/Eastern European countries, 18 Asian countries, 15 countries in the Americas, 10 countries in the Middle East, and 12 countries in Africa. From the data that was collected, the WAO found food allergy cases in preschool children were higher in developed and Westernized countries. In large and rapidly developing societies, such as China, allergy cases appeared to increase as the country became more Westernized. Food allergy cases in Chongqing, China, were observed to double in one- to two-year-olds, from 3.5 percent in 1999 to 7.7 percent in 2009.

Data from the WAO survey identified percentage of the population with food allergies by country as follows:

> For all ages, 0 to 18 years: Australia 6%, China 2%, Japan and Hong Kong 5%, Canada 7%, United States 4 to 8%, Columbia 10 to 13%, Mexico 3%, United Kingdom 16%, Germany 4 to 15%, Switzerland 3%, Greece 5%, Poland 8 to 32%, Netherlands 7 to 26%, Belgium 5%, France 7%, Spain 7 to 10%, Italy 4 to 10%, Turkey 3%, Lithuania 10%, Denmark 3%, Finland 12%, and Morocco 3%.

For children under the age of 5: Australia 10%, China 4 to 8%, Taiwan 3%, Japan 4 to 9%, Hong Kong 5%, Canada 8%, United States 6%, United Kingdom 4 to 6%, France 4%, Norway 7%, Iceland 2%, Sweden 3 to 11%, Finland 9%.

For children 5 and over: Australia 4% (nuts only), Taiwan 8%, Korea 2%, Japan 3 to 5%, Hong Kong 5%, Philippines 2% (fish) to 5% (shellfish), Canada 5%, United States 3%, Columbia 13%, United Kingdom 3%, France 3%, Italy 11%, Turkey 2%, Lithuania 13 to 16%, Denmark 1%, Iceland 16%, Sweden 5%, Israel 4%, United Arab Emirates 8%, Kenya 7%, Ghana 11%, Mozambique 19%, Tanzania 17%, South Africa 5%.

The most common foods that triggered allergy reactions varied by country, and results were as follows:

Australia: cow's milk, egg, peanut, seafood, soy, tree nuts
China: cow's milk, egg, fish, fruit, peanut, shellfish, shrimp
Taiwan: crab, fish, mango, milk, mollusk, peanut, shrimp
Japan: cow's milk, egg, fish, fruit, peanut, shellfish, wheat
Hong Kong: egg, fish, fruits, milk, peanut, shellfish
Philippines: cow's milk, egg, fish, peanut, shellfish, soy
Canada: cow's milk, egg, fish, peanut, seafood, soy, tree nuts, wheat
United States: cow's milk, egg, fish, peanut, seafood, shellfish, soy, tree nuts
Columbia: cow's milk, egg, fruit, meats, seafood, vegetables
Mexico: cacao, chili beans, cow's milk, egg, fish, mango, soy, shrimp, strawberry, wheat
Brazil: corn, cow's milk, egg, fish, peanuts, shellfish, soy, tree nuts, wheat
United Kingdom: cow's milk, egg, fish, peanut, tree nuts
Germany: apple, cow's milk, egg, fish, fruit, peanut, soy, tree nuts, vegetables, wheat
Switzerland: cow's milk, egg, fish, hazelnut, kiwi, peanut, potato, wheat
Greece: cow's milk, egg, fish, fruits, legumes, meats, nuts, shellfish
Netherlands: apple, egg, kiwi, milk, peanuts, pear, tree nuts
France: cow's milk, egg, kiwi, fish, peanuts, shrimp, tree nuts
Spain: beef, cocoa, cow's milk, egg, fish, kiwi, peanut, tree nuts, wheat
Italy: milk, egg, fish, fruits, nuts, vegetables, wheat
Turkey: beef, cocoa, cow's milk, egg, fish, kiwi, peanut, tree nuts, wheat
Denmark: cow's milk, egg, fish, fruits, legumes, nuts, peanut, seafood, soy, vegetables, wheat
Sweden: cow's milk, egg, fish, peanut, soy, tree nuts, wheat
Iceland: cow's milk, egg, fish, peanuts, soy, wheat

Israel: egg, fish, milk, peanut, sesame
United Arab Emirates: cow's milk, egg, fish, fruit, peanut, tree nuts, vegetables, wheat
Ghana: banana, mango, orange, pawpaw, pineapple, peanut
Mozambique: fruits, meats, seafood, vegetables
South Africa: cow's milk, egg, peanut, soy

The WAO concluded that quality record collecting and improved comparative data are urgently needed to determine the actual prevalence of food allergy around the world.

The EuroPrevall Initiative also attempted to determine how many people are affected by food allergies in European countries. Established in 2005, the EuroPrevall Initiative was established by 23 European countries, including Africa and Asia. The EuroPrevall Initiative was a four-year research project that evaluated diet, genetics, and environmental risk factors for individuals with food allergies. Three different study methods were used: a birth cohort study conducted in 9 countries, a general population survey of schoolchildren and adults in 8 countries, and a cross-sectional study of allergy clinics in 12 countries. Birth cohort studies follow people from birth over a specific time period. General population surveys collect data from people within specified geographic boundaries. Cross-sectional studies observe a population at a specific point in time.

The EuroPrevall collected subjective information from individuals who experienced an allergic reaction after eating a food but also confirmed the reaction with skin prick and blood tests and double-blind, placebo-controlled food challenges. This project monitored 12,000 European children. Approximately 37,000 additional children from Russia, China, and India were also added to the study. The study found geographic differences in food allergy prevalence among countries. Preliminary data reports that the United Kingdom, Netherlands, and Lithuania had the highest prevalence of allergy to cow's milk at 1.25 percent of the total population. Greece was found to have the lowest prevalence of allergy to cow's milk and egg and no allergy to peanut. The United Kingdom also had the highest prevalence for egg allergy, 2.2 percent of the population. Overall food allergy prevalence was 2 percent of the population in Hong Kong, 1.04 percent of the population in India, and 0.28–0.67 percent of the population in more rural areas of China. Data from this initiative is still being extrapolated.

Much more data has been collected about peanut allergies in children because of the significant increase of peanut allergy cases in recent decades. Peanut allergies were rare prior to the early 1990s. But by 2008, an estimated 1 percent, or approximately 3 million people, of the U.S. population had a peanut allergy. By 2012, this number was estimated to have increased to about 4 million people. While the incidence of peanut allergies afflicted mostly Western countries in the 1990s, an increase is now being seen in non-Western countries as well. The approximate prevalence of peanut allergy by country, during specified time frames, is as follows:

Table 16.1 World Health Organization Global Survey of Food Allergy Burden in Children

Ghana, Africa	2006	0%
	2013	1.5% and sensitization 17.5%
Australia	1995	0.47%
	2004	1.15%
	2009	2% (approximately 114,400 children)
Montreal, Canada	2007	1.71% under the age of nine years
	2009	1.21–2.33%
Russia	2014	0.08% of children
France	2000	0.45% of children below 15 years
Germany	2005	20% of all food reactions
Hong Kong	2001/2002	Rare
	2008/2009	0.57–1%, ages two to seven
Israel	2002	0.17% Jewish Israeli children
	2012	0.6%, ages 13–14
	2012	2.5%, ages 13–14 Arab Israeli
Japan	2003	Rare
Norway/Denmark	2001	Very low
	2005	0.5% Danish adolescents
Singapore	2007	1.08–1.35%, ages 5–12
Sweden	1998	1.2%
United Kingdom	2007	1.8% school-age children
United States	2002	0.8% below 18 years
	2008	1.4%
	2010	2–2.8%

Source: S. L. Prescott, R. Pawankar, K. J. Allen, D. E. Campbell, J.K.H. Sinn, A. Fiocchi et al. "A Global Survey of Changing Patterns of Food Allergy Burden in Children." *The World Health Organization Journal*, 2013, 6(1): 21.

In summary, it is possible to be allergic to any food in any country. In general, current research finds food allergies occur less often in rural areas than urban areas and in countries that are less developed.

17. Are food allergies and negative reactions to foods on the rise?

Current allergy research is based on self-reported symptoms, and food allergy incidence is estimated by most allergy organizations. Although there is little evidence to verify actual allergy increase in the past few decades, it is generally thought that allergy incidence is rising based on the increased number of allergy patients seen in medical practices and some research. It is also possible that perceived increases may be due to better diagnostic practices.

Few studies have been done about prevalence of food sensitivities and food intolerances. A 2009 study estimated that more than 20 percent of individuals living in industrialized countries had food intolerances. However, little research has been done on food allergy increases. According to the Food Allergy Research & Education organization, food allergies increased approximately 50 percent in children between 1997 and 2011 in the United States. Of these, childhood peanut or tree nut allergies tripled between 1997 and 2008, and food allergies increased 2.1 percent per decade among black children, 1.2 percent per decade among Hispanic children, and 1 percent per decade among white children. The College of Allergy, Asthma and Immunology estimates that peanut allergies has increased 21 percent in children since 2010.

In general, it appears that peanut allergies doubled in Westernized countries around the world between 2005 and 2015. Peanut allergies are also being reported in Africa and Asia for the first time. Over the past decade, no decline in food allergy incidence was seen. Current research also indicates that the amount of time people need to outgrow food allergies has increased when compared to previous generations, indicating an increase in food allergy susceptibility worldwide. An increase in allergy susceptibility was also seen in all countries that implemented the preventative recommendation of avoiding peanuts in the diet of young children until they were older. In 2016 the Imperial College London reported that feeding children peanuts and eggs between the ages of 4 and 11 months of age showed moderate reductions for developing an allergy to these foods. This study evaluated data from 146 independent food allergy studies, but more research is still needed to confirm these results.

Researchers are unsure exactly why food allergies are increasing. Some theories implicate vaccine policies. It is well known that vaccinations manipulate the immune system, changing its normal response. It is also thought that vaccine injections may have unknown effects on the functioning and integrity of the gastrointestinal system. Vaccines contain antigens, stabilizers, adjuvants, preservatives, antibacterials, antifungals, suspending fluids, gels, aborted fetal cells, formaldehyde, and antibiotics along with various other ingredients. The one guaranteed side effect of a vaccine is the production of IgE antibodies.

Dr. Ken Bock posits that thimerosol, a mercury preservative used in vaccines, has a prominent role in increasing the risk for autism, attention deficit hyperactivity disorder, asthma, and allergies, in general. He also stresses the fact that multidose vaccines, which are a number of different vaccines given in one shot at one time, may overwhelm and oversensitize the immune system. However, because an estimated 90 percent of children in the United States have been vaccinated, it is difficult to validate this theory via studies. Research by Tchavdar L. Vassilev in 1978 found aluminum phosphate, used in some vaccines as an adjuvant, stimulates the synthesis of tetanus toxoid–specific anaphylactic and antitoxic antibodies in animal studies. This in turn leads to a prolonged synthesis of IgE antibodies, possibly increasing allergic diseases. A 2000 study did find that episodes of anaphylaxis increased significantly after vaccination.

The concept of homology may also play a factor in vaccine reactions. Homology occurs when two different proteins have the same structure and weight. Also called cross-reactivity, it explains the fact that a person can be allergic to peanuts and tree nuts even though they are from different plant families. The molecular weight of an antigen impacts cross-reactivity reactions. It has been found that lower-weight protein conjugates increase immune reactions better than higher-weight protein conjugates. A conjugate forms when a protein joins with another substance. For example, haemophilus influenza causes bacterial infections that can be severe, especially in infants. Also known as H. influenza type b (Hib), it is a bacterium that also has a polysaccharide capsule containing polyribosyl ribitol phosphate (PRP). Anti-PRP antibodies have a protective effect against infections. When the PRP is purified, it links to other protein carriers and stimulates greater immune reaction. Because of this, Hib proteins are often paired with other viruses, such as diphtheria or tetanus toxins, to increase protection against them. However, these conjugates also have the potential to increase cross-reactivity reactions because Hib proteins are homologous with peanut proteins. A 1980 study found that tetanus and diphtheria bacteria conjugated with Hib produced an increase in

IgE levels and anaphylaxis in children. A 1999 study found pertussis bacteria in vaccines had the potential to induce intestinal hypersensitivity and prolong sensitization to foods in mice because the pertussis bacteria altered intestinal immunity and overstimulated the immune system.

It also appears that countries that paired Hib proteins with the combination vaccine diphtheria, pertussis, and tetanus (DPT) saw an increase in peanut allergies in their countries for the first time. Singapore reported no peanut allergies prior to 2001, when the Hib-DPT vaccine was introduced. By 2007, peanut reactivity cases increased in Singapore. In Tasmania, Australia, no peanut allergies were reported as of 2001 in children aged seven to eight when Tasmania had the lowest vaccinated population in the world. However, in 2001 the Tasmanian government implemented a public health vaccination campaign. By the end of 2001, 94 percent of Tasmanian children were vaccinated, and by 2009 11 percent of Tasmanian children were reported to have peanut allergies.

Because medical science still does not have a complete understanding of vaccination effects over the life span of humans, the U.S. Congress introduced a bill called the Comprehensive Comparative Study of Vaccinated and Unvaccinated Populations Act in 2006, 2007, and 2009 to better understand the health implications of vaccines. These bills did not pass but were reintroduced in 2013 as the Vaccine Safety Study Act. However, this bill has yet to pass, and there have been few studies investigating a possible connection between vaccines and allergy reactions.

Another theory for allergy increase is the increased use of antibiotics for ear infections. From 1988 to 1994, U.S. children had a significant increase in ear infections with a subsequent increase in antibiotic use. A 2013 study discovered that an average of 2.2 antibiotic prescriptions were given to children during the first year of life. This study looked at children born from 2007 to 2009 who were given antibiotics and the impact antibiotics had on the bacterial composition of their gastrointestinal tract. An increased risk for food allergies in children exposed to antibiotics during the first year of life was found. Another study in 1994, which was published in the *Annals of Allergy*, found 86 percent of children who eliminated allergenic foods from their diet had a significant reduction in ear infections. A confirming study found that children who were allergic to dairy had a significant increase in recurring ear infections.

Preservatives and stabilizers used in medications may also play a role in food allergy risk. Refined peanut oil is often used in injectable drugs. The European Food Safety Authority in 2004 investigated the safety of refined peanut oil and concluded that "fully refined peanut oil and fat" in food and medications could cause allergic reactions in peanut-allergic individuals. It subsequently required that peanut oil used in a product must be included on its label. The U.S. Food and Drug Administration (FDA) also noted trace peanut proteins are found in refined oils. However, it did not prohibit its use nor make labeling mandatory. Labeling oils in the United States in injectable drugs continues to be voluntary, although the FDA does acknowledge that ingredients with increased toxic effects should be noted in contraindications, warning, or precaution sections of the drug label.

Treatment of Food Allergies, Intolerances, and Sensitivities and Prevention

18. How are food allergies treated?

The first line of defense for treating food allergies is to avoid the trigger food or foods. This means reading food labels, asking how meals or foods are prepared when eating away from home, and being very careful about every food that is eaten. However, there are times when, despite best efforts, an allergic reaction does occur. Because of this it is always recommended that an individual with food allergies always wear a medical alert bracelet. Treatment is varied and will depend on the symptoms a person has when having a reaction.

The most severe food allergy reaction is anaphylaxis, which is life threatening. Anaphylaxis is an immune response that affects the respiratory system, causing difficulty breathing or swelling of the throat. It is critical that those individuals susceptible to anaphylaxis and their caregivers recognize the early symptoms of a reaction and respond immediately with self-treatment. Anaphylaxis can be and is usually fatal without emergency treatment. Emergency medications for severe allergy reactions contain epinephrine, and follow-up medical care should then be sought as quickly as possible.

However, individuals do not always experience anaphylaxis. Some may only have hives, vomiting, or abdominal pain, to name a few. But these symptoms can progress to anaphylaxis over the short time span of a few hours. An individual should always be monitored carefully for any change in symptoms after initial self-treatment is given. It is often recommended that the individual go to the emergency room for observation, even if symptoms are mild.

Sometimes an allergenic food, which usually causes a reaction, may be eaten without any symptoms occurring. When this happens, the individual's physician should be contacted immediately and the person transported to the emergency room, even if symptoms are not present. Over-the-counter medications, such as Benadryl®, can also be administered for mild reactions when an EpiPen, which contains epinephrine, is unavailable or the person has a history of mild reactions that do not require further intervention. Immediate medical care continues to be advised after administering self-treatment options for mild reactions. Milder reactions that involve the skin often resolve with topical or oral antihistamines.

Anti-IgE therapy has been used with some success in food allergy treatment. Because most severe food allergies with rapid onset of symptoms are triggered by the production of the immunoglobulin IgE, anti-IgE therapies have been tried to reduce or eliminate an allergic reaction. Anti-IgE therapy uses a medicine that contains an antibody that binds with IgE in the bloodstream and is injected once per week for two to four weeks. The theory behind this therapy is that the medicine reduces the amount of IgE antibodies in the bloodstream, thus reducing or eliminating an allergic reaction. Anti-IgE therapy has been successfully used in some asthma patients who do not respond well to other treatments. It has been tried with food allergy patients with some success; however, not all individuals experience improvement, and the degree of improvement varies from person to person. The treatment itself may also cause an allergic reaction.

Other potential therapies that have been used with some success include herbal therapies and probiotics. Chinese herbal therapies have been used for centuries to treat allergy reactions. Dr. Xiu-Min Li at Jaffe Food Allergy Institute at Mount Sinai uses a traditional Chinese medicine formulary tailored to allergy symptoms, which has been effective in mice with peanut allergy. However, more research is still needed in this area. Using probiotics has also been tried because the hygiene hypothesis suggests that an overactive immune system may be looking for something to "fight" in the absence of everyday germs to keep itself "busy." Because of this hypothesis, it is thought that healthy bacteria in the gastrointestinal tract may make the immune system less likely to attack harmless proteins found in food. Probiotics, in general, provide a safe way to balance bacteria in the gastrointestinal tract, although individuals with a compromised immune system or who have liver conditions should not take probiotics due to an increased risk for fatal infections. Study results regarding probiotic effectiveness for treating food allergies have been poor, but research continues in this area.

19. How are food intolerances treated?

Food intolerance reactions are rarely life threatening or require medications for their treatment. They do not provoke a histamine response by the immune system, unlike food allergies. Small amounts of an offending food also do not tend to cause symptoms, as they would in food allergy. Frequently, symptoms can occur within several hours or up to 48 hours after eating the food. Symptoms can also last for days until they improve or resolve. Therefore, it is more important to determine what foods are causing symptoms and avoid them in the diet at all times. But as with food allergies, accidental ingestion of offending foods can occur.

The majority of food intolerances affect the gastrointestinal system. Treatment depends on individual symptoms. Abdominal pain, stomachaches, bloating, cough, gas, headaches or migraines, hives, and runny nose will usually resolve over a period of time after the suspected food is eliminated from the diet. Irritable bowel symptoms may also resolve after the suspected food is eliminated from the diet. However, some over-the-counter medications that are effective for specific symptoms may help control them until they resolve. For example, for diarrhea the over-the-counter drug Imodium® can be given for short-term control.

The most important strategy to limit or prevent food intolerance symptoms is to read food labels and ask how foods are cooked when eating away from home. It is especially critical to be familiar with different ingredient names that indicate a potential allergenic food. Ingredient names for the most common intolerances are as follows.

Other ingredient names for milk and lactose are anhydrous milk fat, butter, casein and caseinates, cheese, cream, curds, custard, dairy product solids, galactose, ghee, half and half, hydrolysates, ice cream, ice milk, lactalbumin, lactalbumin phosphate, lactate solids, lactitol monohydrate, lactoglobulin, lactulose, lactic acid yeast, milk fat, nisin preparation, nougat, pudding, quark, recaldent, rennet, rennet casein, sherbet, simplesse, sour cream—solids and imitation, whey, whipped cream, yogurt, and yogurt powder.

Other ingredient names for gluten are barley, brewer's yeast, durum, Einkorn wheat, emmer, farina, faro, graham, kamut khorasan wheat, malt, rye, semolina, spelt, triticale, wheat, wheat starch, and wheat berries.

Other ingredient names for fructose include high-fructose corn syrup, corn syrup, the sugar alcohols sorbitol, isomalt, lactitol, maltitol, mannitol, xylitol, erythritol, hydrogenated starch hydrolysates, agave nectar, barley malt, crystalline fructose, high-fructose fruit (apple, banana, blackberry, blueberries, cherry, dried fruits, fig, grapes, kiwi, lychee, mandarin, mango, star fruit, rock melon, grapefruit, pear, pineapple, pomegranate, quince, raspberries, tomato concentrate), fruit juice concentrate, glucose syrup, honey, maize syrup, rice syrup, and tapioca syrup.

Other ingredient names for soy are bean curd, edamame, hydrolyzed plant protein, hydrolyzed soy protein, hydrolyzed vegetable protein, kinnoko flour, miso, natto, natural flavoring, okara, shoyu sauce, soy lecithin, soya flour, soybeans, supro, syodofu, tamatri, tempeh, teriyaki sauce, textured soy flour protein, textured vegetable protein, tofu, vegetable broth, vegetable gum, vegetable starch, yakidofu, and yuba (bean curd).

Other ingredient names for sulfites include caustic sulfite caramel, calcium sulfite, calcium hydrogen sulfite, sulfur dioxide, potassium hydrogen sulfite, sulfite ammonia caramel, potassium bisulfite, sulfite, or metabisulfite, sodium bisulfite, metabisulfite, sulfite, and sulfur dioxide.

Other ingredient names for peanuts are arachic oil, arachis, arachis hypogaea, artificial nuts, beer, earth, or ground nuts, goobers or goober peas, hydrolyzed peanut protein, hypogaeic acid, mandelonas, mixed nuts, monkey nuts, nu nuts, and nutmeat.

Other ingredient names for tree nuts are almond, beechnut, Brazil nut, bush nut, butternut, cashew, chestnut, filbert, ginko fruit, hazelnut, hickory nut, lichee nut, macadamia nut, nangai nut, pecan, pine nut, pistachio, shea nut, and walnut.

Other ingredient names for eggs include albumin, apovitellin, cholesterol-free egg substitute, dried egg solids, egg white, egg wash, eggnog, fat substitutes, globulin, lecithin, livetin, lysozyme, mayonnaise, meringue, ovalbumin, ovomucin, ovotransferrin, ovovitella, powdered eggs, silici albuminate, simplesse, surimi, trailblazer, and vitellin.

20. How are food sensitivities treated?

As with food allergies and food intolerances, eliminating the allergenic food in the diet is the primary treatment for all food sensitivities. However, unlike food intolerance, some food sensitivities can involve the immune system and become life threatening. As discussed previously, medically recognized abnormal reactions to food that are classified as food sensitivities are gluten-sensitive enteropathy (celiac disease), food-dependent, exercise-induced anaphylaxis, allergic eosinophilic gastroenteritis, food protein–induced enterocolitis syndrome, food protein–induced proctocolitis, oral allergy syndrome, sulfite-induced asthma, and leaky gut. While avoiding the trigger food or foods in the daily diet is critical to prevent a reaction, each condition has its own treatment plan should an allergic reaction occur.

Following a strict gluten-free diet is the primary treatment for gluten-sensitive enteropathy (celiac sprue) and non-celiac gluten sensitivity. When gluten is eliminated from the diet, the villi begin to heal, eventually resuming their ability to absorb nutrients. Symptoms usually resolve once the villi are healed. A small percentage of celiac patients who do not improve with a gluten-free diet may need corticosteroid medications to improve and manage their symptoms.

Treatment for food-dependent, exercise-induced anaphylaxis (FDEIA) eliminates trigger foods from the diet before or after exercise. Eating any meal or snack at least four hours, which allows for complete digestion, before exercise and avoiding alcohol, aspirin, or nonsteroidal anti-inflammatory drugs before exercise may reduce or eliminate a reaction. It is also recommended to individuals diagnosed with FDEIA that injectable epinephrine (e.g., EpiPen) be carried with them whenever they are exercising. It is recommended that a medical alert bracelet be worn.

Treatment for allergic eosinophilic gastroenteritis involves eliminating eggs, fish, milk, peanuts, shellfish, soy, tree nuts, and wheat from the diet for at least six weeks since these foods are known to trigger most eosinophilic symptoms. Sometimes all foods are eliminated, and the individual is put on an elemental diet. Elemental diets are liquid diets made of easily absorbed nutrients essential for health. Steroid and anti-inflammatory medications as well as nutrition supplements may also be prescribed. An absolute eosinophil count (blood test) is checked after six weeks, and the treatment plan is reevaluated and adjusted depending on test results and symptom management.

Treatment for food protein–induced enterocolitis syndrome (FPIES) includes emergency intravenous hydration because of the increased risk for rapid dehydration and shock during acute reactions. Children with severe reactions benefit from steroids and hospitalization. Hypoallergenic or elemental baby formulas or breastfeeding may eliminate symptoms of FPIES in infants. For those with few food sensitivities that trigger FPIES, avoiding the trigger food(s) in the diet may be all that is needed. As a child grows, food challenges will be given to monitor tolerance as most children outgrow FPIES. FPIES in adults is usually permanent.

Food-induced proctocolitis treatment requires eliminating all trigger foods from the diet, including in the mother's diet if she is breastfeeding. An elimination diet is used to determine which food or foods the infant is sensitive to.

Treatment for oral allergy syndrome varies, depending on individual pollen allergies. However, avoiding trigger foods is critical. For those who experience severe symptoms, it is recommended that an adrenaline auto-injector be carried at all times. Some oral allergy syndrome patients are able to eat trigger foods that are cooked, avoiding all raw forms of the suspected food. Specific pollen allergens are also found in foods. The most common seasonal allergens and their potential raw food counterparts are as follows:

Birch allergies: raw almonds, apples, apricots, carrots, coriander, celery, cherries, fennel, hazelnuts, kiwi, nectarines, parsnips, peaches, pears, peppers, and plums.

Ragweed allergies: raw bananas, cantaloupe, chamomile tea, cucumber, honeydew, sunflower seeds, watermelon, and zucchini.

Grass allergies: celery, cantaloupe, honeydew, oranges, peaches, tomatoes, and watermelon.

Mugwort allergies: raw apples, bell peppers, black pepper, broccoli, cabbage, caraway, carrots, celery, coriander, fennel, kiwi, parsley, peanuts, and sunflowers.

Latex allergies: raw avocados, bananas, chestnuts, kiwi, and papaya.

While these are foods that may trigger symptoms because their protein component closely matches the protein component found in these pollens, not all foods listed will. Some people experience symptoms after eating only one or two of these foods but no symptoms after eating other high-risk foods. Following an elimination diet is usually recommended to patients with oral allergy syndrome to determine high-risk foods.

Treatment for sulfite-induced asthma includes avoiding all foods with added or naturally occurring sulfites and carrying an adrenaline auto-injector, such as an EpiPen.

Treatment for leaky gut will depend on individual symptoms. In general, all foods or food components (food dyes, preservatives, etc.) that trigger sensitivity reactions must be eliminated from the daily diet. Gluten-free and dairy-free diets are also recommended as possible triggers of inflammation in the intestine. If the root cause of leaky gut symptoms is antibiotic use or a virus, rebalancing the gut with beneficial probiotics and eating foods that help heal the gastrointestinal system, such as bone broth and fermented foods, may resolve leaky gut symptoms. A knowledgeable medical professional may also prescribe other specific dietary supplements that are known to heal the gastrointestinal tract, such as glutathione or slippery elm, after an evaluation.

21. What is an emergency treatment plan for severe allergic reactions?

Anyone with a food allergy, and their caregivers, should always carry a written emergency treatment plan and emergency care kit with them. It is essential to recognize the early symptoms of a food allergy reaction and immediately begin self-treatment. Emergency medical care should then be sought as soon as possible.

A food allergy action plan should always include a list of foods that the individual is allergic to, a list of symptoms that can potentially occur, a list of prescribed medications and doses, a list of steps to follow during a reaction, names and phone numbers of emergency contacts (minimum of three), names and phone numbers of doctors and hospitals, and a written summary from the individual's doctor outlining medical history and suggested treatment plan during an emergency. The Food Allergy and Anaphylaxis Network provides a sample copy of the information that should be included in a food allergy action plan on its website.

An emergency care kit should also be ready for use and available at all times. This kit should include lifesaving medications that are prescribed to the individual by his or her physician and the food allergy action plan. All friends, family, teachers, and coworkers should be instructed on how to administer the medications prescribed. A list of action steps to be followed during an emergency should also be kept in the kit in the event a stranger must administer medications.

Emergency medications for allergy reactions contain epinephrine. Epinephrine is a hormone produced by the adrenal glands and is also known as adrenaline. It is derived from the amino acid tyrosine and typically produced in response to the fight or flight response that occurs during threatening situations. Administering epinephrine opens up airways to ease breathing and narrows blood vessels to raise blood pressure, which reduces the risk of fainting.

The most commonly prescribed epinephrine medication is an EpiPen. The EpiPen was introduced in the 1980s and is an auto-injector device that administers the correct dose of epinephrine to the individual, halting the histamine response to an allergen and slowing the allergic reaction. It also relaxes muscles and eases breathing. An EpiPen is easy to use and the quickest way to administer lifesaving medication because it provides one measured dose. Mylan Pharmaceutical provides a short video on its website instructing people how to administer an EpiPen correctly. There are other brands of single-dose epinephrine medications available to patients as well.

Epinephrine should be injected in the middle of the outer thigh while holding the leg firmly in place before and during the injection. Injecting it into the thigh facilitates the circulation of epinephrine into the bloodstream, quickly stopping anaphylaxis. It can be injected through clothing if necessary during an emergency. It should never be injected into the buttocks or any other part of the body because it takes longer to get into the circulation. There will be some liquid that remains in the auto-injector after administration. This is normal and does not mean the correct dose was not given. The extra liquid should be disposed of properly and not injected. If epinephrine is accidentally injected, emergency medical treatment should be sought immediately.

In general, symptoms begin to lessen after administration of epinephrine. However, if symptoms have not improved after 10 minutes, a second injection of epinephrine is advised. Most auto-injectors contain only one dose of epinephrine, so two auto-injectors should always be included in the emergency kit. After epinephrine is administered, the individual should be transported to the nearest emergency room for observation because epinephrine has a short half-life, which means symptom relief is only temporary. More than two injections of epinephrine should be administered only by a health-care professional.

Food allergy action plans and emergency kits should always be checked and updated at least annually or whenever there is a change in medical condition or medications. Medication expiration dates should also be checked and medications replaced as needed, even if rarely used. In an emergency, money spent on replacement medications may mean the difference between life and death and is well worth the replacement cost.

Wearing a medical alert bracelet at all times to identify the potential allergy during a medical emergency if unable to respond to questions is advised. The MedicAlert Foundation provides medical alert jewelry, although there are many other companies available that provide this service.

22. What are the pros and cons of banning allergenic foods from schools or public places?

According to the American College of Allergy, Asthma and Immunology, peanut allergies in children have increased 21 percent since 2010, and an estimated 8 percent of children are allergic to one or more foods. Because so many more children have food allergies than ever before, schools, day cares, and other public places where children congregate have struggled to manage the number of children with food allergies who enter their facilities daily. The most common solution for many of these public facilities has been to ban peanuts and nuts, with other food allergies addressed case by case because of their rarity. But there are pros and cons to banning allergenic foods.

The primary goal of banning allergenic foods is to keep children and adults safe from potential food allergy reactions. Two approaches to achieve this goal is allergen avoidance and training programs designed to prepare staff to appropriately treat an allergic reaction should it occur. The most popular approach taken to keep students safe is to ban peanuts and nuts in schools and most public places, which was started in the 1990s. Supporters of peanut and nut bans believed that this would decrease the risk for accidental peanut exposure and also reduce the anxiety and social stigma that some of those with food allergies feel when away from home. "Safe" tables, a table specifically for those with food allergies, are set up in a designated area to minimize risk of peanut or nut allergy exposures.

However, opponents to a peanut and nut ban argue that peanut bans are difficult to enforce and do not eliminate 100 percent of the risk, leading to a false sense of security that may actually increase risk for an allergy reaction. In addition, those without peanut/nut allergies are forced to give up foods they like and may feel deprived of a favorite food or not eat well because they eat only peanut butter. It is also argued that the allergenic child may feel singled out, especially if he or she must sit at a peanut- or nut-free lunch table, or be bullied by others because he or she is different. An unintended consequence may also expose children with other food allergies than nuts, increasing their risk for an allergy reaction since their needs are often not considered in setting up nut- and peanut-free zones.

Both proponents and opponents of peanut and nut bans need to consider if peanut and nut allergens are actually detected and, if so, how much is detected and how great the risk to children really is. One 2004 study by Perry, Conover-Walker, Pomes, Chapman, and Wood found that peanut allergens were detectable on cafeteria tables, desktops, water faucets, and food preparation areas in the sample schools studied. However, the level detected was 130 nanogram (ng)/milliliter (ml). This level of allergen exposure was unlikely to elicit an allergic reaction. Objective studies find that doses in the 2- to 50-milligram (mg) range triggered allergic reactions; 130 ng is equivalent to 0.00013 mg, which is far below the trigger range. This study concluded that traditional cleaning methods used to clean tables and other common objects were just as effective for peanut allergen removal and decreasing the risk for allergenic reactions as banning peanuts.

Another consideration is how many food allergy reactions occur in the school setting. Studies in the United States and the United Kingdom have shown that approximately 3.1–14.3 percent of school-age children experienced a peanut or tree nut allergy reaction. However, the majority of these reactions occurred in the child's home or at a friend's or relative's house. Studies specifically exploring the effectiveness of peanut bans in public settings have yet to be done, but some general studies exploring peanut allergy incidence give us an idea. Studies by Nguyen-Lu et al. in 2012 found that 15 percent of children with food allergies experienced accidental exposures. Of these, 40 percent occurred in their home, 17 percent occurred at the home of a friend or relative, and 6 percent occurred in the school setting. Of those that occurred at school, 71 percent occurred in schools that banned peanuts and 29 percent occurred in schools that did not ban peanuts. Another study found that accidental peanut exposure was actually greater in schools with peanut restrictions than in those that did not ban them.

Even with peanut and nut bans, it is impossible to remove the risk of being exposed to an allergen 100 percent, and enforcement of peanut-/nut-free zones is difficult. It is always possible that another food may be present at lunches and snacks that was processed in a plant that also processes nuts or peanuts, so trace contamination remains possible. One study that looked at schools with peanut bans found that even when parents were notified and educated about the peanut ban, 0.6 percent of home lunches still contained peanuts. Therefore, it is argued that a peanut ban can provide a false sense of security, making the allergenic child, parents, and staff less cautious and aware of the possibility of peanuts being present. While there is no evidence to date that banning peanuts and nuts in school prevents fatal or near-fatal allergic reactions, it has been found in a few studies that delayed use of epinephrine was the major cause of fatality. Therefore, the emphasis on education and training about food allergies and proper treatment of allergy reactions was actually more important than banning the offending food.

Dr. Julie Wang and Dr. David M. Fleischer endorse more effective strategies that suggest parents and guardians be the only people to provide food and snacks for their allergenic child. They also recommend allergy-friendly cafeterias with increased supervision and careful and routine cleaning of toys, tables, desktops, or other commonly shared objects with soap and water or commercial wipes. Foods should always be properly labeled with the name of the child, and food allergens should be avoided in crafts, science, or cooking projects. Alternative ingredients could also be supplied or an alternate activity planned for the allergenic child if the project is risky. Staff should be regularly trained on recognition and management of allergy reactions, and written emergency action plans, including photos, should be readily accessible. The facility should have a standard written policy for food allergy management and regular training programs for staff and caregivers.

Managing Nutrition and Food Reactions in the Real World

23. How does an individual stay healthy and manage their diet when one or more food groups must be eliminated from the daily diet?

Eliminating any food group from the daily diet can be problematic. Every food group has nutritional benefits. The six main food groups that are important for good health are dairy, fats, fruits, grains, proteins, and vegetables. To understand the impact of eliminating any one food group, it is essential to understand how each one functions.

Nutrition is the science that studies the impact food has on the growth, development, and health of the human body. Food, in the proper amounts and balance, provides energy and essential nutrients for survival and good health. Numerous studies have also verified that optimal nutrient intakes during the development, growth, and future health of a child are crucial. While there are numerous beneficial substances in foods, the most important food nutrients are classified as macronutrients, micronutrients, antioxidants, and water.

Macronutrients provide energy that makes the body run and are classified as carbohydrates, proteins, and fats. Each macronutrient has a specific function. Carbohydrates fuel the body, providing energy in the form of calories. There are two types of carbohydrates: simple and complex. Simple carbohydrates require little digestion and supply a fast, usable energy source. Simple carbohydrate sources include all forms of table sugars, corn syrup and high-fructose corn syrup, fruit juice, honey, maple syrup, soda, white bread, white rice and pasta, and most cereals and baked goods. Complex carbohydrates require more time and effort to break down into a form the body can use for energy and to provide fiber that supports the removal of waste from the gastrointestinal tract after digestion. Fiber is a natural substance found in plant foods such as legumes, vegetables, and whole grains and is made up of different fibers. But fiber's importance is primarily for the health and normal functioning of the gastrointestinal system. A well-functioning gastrointestinal tract can significantly impact vitamin and mineral production and absorption as well as the manufacturing of hormones and enzymes.

Complex carbohydrate sources include fruit, grains such as quinoa, legumes, starchy vegetables such as corn, peas, potato, sweet potato, vegetables, winter squash, whole grains such as brown rice, whole grain pasta and cereals, and whole wheat breads.

Protein supplies energy in the form of calories, but its primary role is to provide building blocks, called amino acids. Amino acids are necessary for growth, repair, and maintenance of body tissues and muscles. Proteins also support the immune system's ability to fight infections, support decreased inflammation, and are critical for fetal growth and development. Protein sources include eggs, fish, some dairy foods, legumes, poultry, pork, red meat, and soybeans. Fats, also known as lipids, are important sources of fatty acids and supply energy in the form of calories. Fatty acids are necessary to absorb fat-soluble vitamins and are used in many biological processes throughout the body. Research shows that "healthy" fats are critical for the formation of the brain, eyes, and nervous system during fetal growth. Fatty acids are also essential for growth and good health throughout the life cycle. There are two types of fatty acids: essential and nonessential fatty acids. Essential fatty acids are important for brain function, skin and joint health, hair growth, metabolism, and heart health. They are not manufactured by the body and must be eaten from food sources. The body also produces nonessential fatty acids when it needs them; therefore, these fatty acids are not required from the foods we eat.

Fats are further classified into saturated and unsaturated categories. Unsaturated fats are broken down into monounsaturated and polyunsaturated categories. Saturated fats are known as "bad" fats. These are the fats that are typically solid at room temperature and implicated in developing heart disease as we age. Although new research indicates that saturated fats may not be as bad as first thought, it is still recommended that these fats be eaten in moderation. Trans fats are a subclass of saturated fats. *Trans fats* are synthesized during a chemical process that hydrogenates oils, which increases the shelf life of a food. Hydrogenated oils are found mainly in margarines; shortening; and processed foods such as crackers, cookies, French fries, baked goods, microwave popcorn, and cream-filled candies. They act like saturated fats in the body, having a negative effect on heart health. Butterfat, meats, lamb, and dairy products have naturally occurring trans fats, but studies have not yet shown if these naturally occurring trans fats have the same negative impact as man-made trans fats. Food sources of saturated fats include butter, cheese, coconut, ice cream and other dairy desserts, whole fat milk, yogurt; most cookies and baked goods; bacon, deli and processed meats, red meats, sausage; pizza and other fast-food meals; and most processed foods.

Unsaturated fats are known as "healthy" fats and have been shown to protect the cardiovascular system, brain, and joints and to reduce inflammation. They are found mostly in plant foods. A further categorization of unsaturated fats includes monounsaturated fats found in avocados and avocado oil; olive, peanut and canola oils; nuts (almonds, hazelnuts, pecans); and pumpkin, sesame, and sunflower seeds. Polyunsaturated fats are found in corn, sunflower, soybean, and flaxseed oils; flax seeds and walnuts; and fatty, cold-water fishes (black cod, blue fish, herring, mackerel, salmon, sardines, sea bass, swordfish, tuna). One important nutritional distinction among essential fatty acids are linoleic, linolenic, and alpha-linoleic fatty acids, also known as Omega-3, 6, and 9 fatty acids. Omega-3s and Omega-6s are found in polyunsaturated fats and are not synthesized by the body. This means they must be eaten in the daily diet and are considered essential for good health. Omega-9s are found in monounsaturated fats and are synthesized within the body when needed, therefore making them nonessential.

The most important of the three omega fatty acids is Omega-3 fatty acids, which are an integral part of cell membrane structures and involved in many crucial biochemical pathways within the body. They are necessary for synthesis of hormones and enzymes, are anti-inflammatory, and overall have been found to be essential in the prevention of many diseases as we age. They are synthesized from linolenic acid found in fish. They are further converted into eicosapentaenoic acid (EPA) and docosahexaenonic acid (DHA). There is also a plant-based source of Omega-3s known as alpha-linolenic acid (ALA). ALA is found in flax seeds, chia seeds, and walnuts. While plant sources will also convert into DHA and EPA, its conversion is less efficient and considered a suboptimal form of EPA and DHA. Fish and marine fish oils are currently considered the best source for Omega-3s. Food sources of *Omega-3s* include fish, marine fish oils, flax seeds and flaxseed oil, grass-fed animals, walnuts, and canola and soybean oils.

Micronutrients are commonly known as vitamins and minerals and act as cofactors in biological processes essential for normal growth, metabolism, and health. Vitamins and minerals are the "spark plugs" that ignite your "fuel," controlling the critical functions used by the body to make your engine "run" smoothly and efficiently. Suboptimal intake of essential micronutrients will result in poor health and chronic illnesses. Micronutrients are just as important as macronutrients for good health.

Vitamins are essential organic nutrients used for energy and as cofactors in many different biochemical reactions. Vitamins support bone formation, enzyme and hormone production, eye and skin health, immunity, metabolism, and wound healing among many other functions. They must come from food sources and are usually needed only in small amounts by healthy individuals.

Minerals are inorganic nutrients that are just as involved in biochemical processes as vitamins. They too are needed in minute amounts by healthy individuals and play a supporting role in growth and maintaining health. Antioxidants, also called phytonutrients, are a more recent nutrient classification. They are "helpers and protectors" found in certain plant foods, especially in fruits and vegetables. More than 25,000 phytochemicals have been discovered in plant foods. While many of their benefits are still being studied, we do know that carotenoids, ellagic acid, flavonoids, glucosinolates, phytoestrogens, and resveratrol have potential positive health impacts and are necessary for optimal health.

Vitamins are classified as fat-soluble and water-soluble vitamins. Fat-soluble vitamins must be paired with fats in foods for optimal absorption. These vitamins are also stored by the body in the liver and fat tissue if they are not needed. Therefore, daily dietary intake of these nutrients is not necessary for most people. If these vitamins are consumed in large quantities over time, either by food or supplement, it is possible for a person to become toxic with negative health outcomes.

Water-soluble vitamins are absorbed without additional macronutrient support and removed by the body (usually by the kidneys) if they are overconsumed. Excessive amounts of a water-soluble vitamin over a long period of time may cause a negative health consequence, but this is extremely rare. For example, there is a condition known as carotenemia. Carotenemia occurs when foods or dietary supplements high in beta carotene (the precursor of vitamin A) are overeaten, such as carrots, winter squash, and sweet potatoes. The first symptom of carotenemia involves the skin and whites of the eyes, which turns yellow or orange. However, if sources of carotene are avoided, the person returns to normal.

Fat-soluble vitamins are A, D, E, and K. Water-soluble vitamins are thiamine, riboflavin, niacin, pantothenic acid, vitamin B_6, folic acid, vitamin B_{12}, biotin, vitamin C, and choline.

Minerals, like vitamins, are used to support the health of bones, muscles, the heart, and brain and used as cofactors in biochemical reactions and enzyme and hormone production. There are two classes of minerals: macrominerals and trace minerals. Macrominerals are required by the body in larger amounts than trace minerals, to maintain good health. Macrominerals are calcium, chloride, magnesium, phosphorus, potassium, and sodium. Trace minerals are copper, fluoride, iodine, iron, manganese, nickel, selenium, and zinc.

Water is also classified as an essential nutrient because all biochemical reactions occur in water. It is required for digestion, absorption, and transport of nutrients and removal of waste products. Without water, death occurs within three days (although some people have survived as many as eight days). Water makes up 50–80 percent of the body, and dehydration of 2 percent of body weight significantly impairs performance and bodily functions.

As the result of years of research, the Institute of Medicine established minimum and maximum recommended daily dietary amounts for each vitamin and mineral. These are known as dietary reference intakes (DRIs). DRIs include information from the recommended dietary allowances, adequate intakes, and tolerable upper intake level based on available evidence and scientific judgment. These values are formulated for healthy individuals. Individuals with chronic or compromised health conditions may require additional amounts.

As can be seen, eliminating any one food group or food category can have a significant impact on health as all food groups and their nutritional benefits are interconnected. Eliminating one or more food allergen groups can cause vitamin or mineral deficiencies, weight loss or gain, anxiety, or increased calorie needs to repair the skin or gastrointestinal system if inflammation of the intestines or severe skin rashes occur.

Common food allergens eliminated from the diet may cause the following potential nutrient deficiencies:

Eggs: pantothenic acid, riboflavin, vitamin B_{12}, selenium
Milk: calcium, pantothenic acid, phosphorus, riboflavin, vitamin A, vitamin D, vitamin B_{12}

Peanut: chromium, magnesium, manganese, niacin, vitamin E
Soy: folate, iron, magnesium, phosphorus, riboflavin, thiamin, zinc
Tree nuts: magnesium, selenium
Wheat: iron, niacin, riboflavin, thiamin

The most effective strategy to ensure the daily diet of an allergenic individual adequately meets his or her nutritional needs is to meet with an experienced health professional who specializes in nutrition and food allergies, such as a registered dietitian (RD). RDs or registered dietitian nutritionists (RDNs) are health-care professionals who receive a bachelor's degree studying food and nutrition, complete an accredited and supervised nutrition practice program, and pass a national certification exam to become RDs. To maintain their certification as nutrition specialists, they are required to complete continuing education programs throughout their career. Many RDs or RDNs specialize in food allergies and food sensitivities and offer specialized testing and diet planning evaluating them. Meeting with an RD or RDN includes a review of diet habits and eating patterns, analysis of nutrient intake, identification of potential deficiencies, and the formation of a specific and individualized diet plan to meet daily nutrition needs that avoids allergenic foods but supplies missing nutrients in alternative foods. Sometimes the use of dietary supplements may be necessary.

24. Can an individual eat out in restaurants, at school, or in public places without fear?

Yes, an individual can. But every precaution to ensure allergen avoidance and appropriate emergency treatment availability are always necessary. Every social and educational setting or meal/snack presents potential dangers. It is impossible to avoid potential allergen exposures in public settings, despite the most stringent precautions taken to avoid allergen exposure. Many individuals who have food allergies find these situations to be time consuming to plan and anxiety provoking. In addition, the individual with the food allergy is not perceived to be "ill" or to have a serious health condition by others, so meal preparation is not always taken as seriously as it should be.

The most common mistakes individuals make when eating away from home involves assuming a food is safe to eat or not being aware of possible cross contamination of foods that are usually safe to eat. Cross contamination occurs when an allergenic food comes into contact with a usually safe food. For some individuals, even the smallest contact between the foods can cause an allergic reaction. This is one reason why label reading is essential for safety. Food manufacturers are required to identify if their food product is processed in a facility that also processes potentially allergenic foods, such as eggs, milk, nuts, peanuts, or wheat.

The best strategy to avoid a reaction is to be proactive. Educating family members, friends, restaurant waitstaff, and teachers about the potential risk for a food allergy reaction is crucial. Having an food allergy action plan and emergency care kit always available, while also educating others about what to do before a food allergy reaction occurs is critical for safety. Employees in restaurants, fast-food establishments, and health-care kitchens are required to receive training about food allergies, how to prevent cross-contamination dangers, and how to administer emergency care should an exposure occur. Restaurants and schools should also ensure that all counters, tables, and utensils are thoroughly cleaned and sanitized with approved cleaning products to minimize food allergens and the possibility of a cross-contamination exposure of an allergenic food.

When eating out in a restaurant, anyone with a food allergy should always ask if a separate food preparation area is used for special diets, if separate cutting boards and utensils are used to prepare special meals, if allergen-free grilled or fried foods share the same grill or fryolator oil as regular meals, who is preparing the meal and if they are juggling numerous meals that can possibly increase a cross-contamination exposure or mistake, how the meal will be labeled and served, and if tables are sanitized between guests. Similar questions can be asked of their host when eating at a friend's house or family gathering.

25. How does an allergic individual navigate the supermarket safely?

Label reading for those with food allergies and their caregivers is a crucial survival skill when shopping for food in the supermarket. Most people assume that if a product does not have an allergen listed on the label, it is safe to eat. However, this is not always the case nor safe. Even though an allergenic food may not be listed on the label, the food item could still be processed in a facility where allergenic foods are manufactured. This increases the risk for a cross contamination between foods and an allergic reaction.

In the United States, the Food Allergen Labeling and Consumer Protection Act (FALCPA) became effective January 1, 2006. This federal government regulation requires that foods that contain major food allergens (eggs, fish, milk, peanuts, shellfish, soy, tree nuts, and wheat) be labeled in an easy-to-understand and noticeable way so that the consumer is aware of the allergen in the food. FALCPA also requires the ingredient be listed in its common name rather than its scientific name.

In the United States, food manufacturers use Good Manufacturing Practices (GMPs) to process foods for sale to the public, in restaurants, and at health-care facilities. GMPs require complete cleaning and sanitation of food processing machinery between uses and the scheduling of specific times to produce nonallergenic food products if applicable. However, even with these precautions in place, there is always a possibility of unintentional contamination with an allergenic ingredient unless the facility is dedicated to nonallergenic food production.

Cross contamination, also called cross contact, occurs when a small amount of a food allergen accidentally gets onto another food that does not have allergens. This can happen in a food manufacturing facility that processes both nonallergenic and allergenic foods together via air contamination. For example, peanut "dust" may be circulating in the air during processing and settle on the nonallergenic food being processed. Also, inadequate cleaning and sanitation of manufacturing equipment between food production items may leave allergen particles that are transferred to the nonallergenic food during processing. The FALCPA does not require food manufacturers to list if cross contamination is possible, but anyone purchasing a food product must be aware of this possibility if they live with or care for someone with a food allergy.

There are differences between countries on how much information is supplied on a food label. In the United States, food manufacturers use the 2 percent rule, which means ingredients are listed on the label only if they are above 2 percent of the total weight of the food product. While this rule protects the proprietary nature of the food manufacturers, thus protecting their "secret" ingredients, it can prove to be a problem for those with food allergies, sensitivities, or intolerances. As a result the FALCPA requires that food allergen ingredients be listed on the label, even if they fall under the 2 percent rule and would otherwise be exempt. Food labels in Australia, Canada, Western Europe, and New Zealand are very strictly regulated and list all ingredients and allergens, regardless of the amount of ingredient present.

While laws require the listing of the eight major allergens on food labels, those who struggle with gluten or other food sensitivities may have a more difficult time finding products that will not affect them. Many food manufacturers in the United States voluntarily list advisory statements on food labels if their food product is at risk for cross contamination because of increased consumer demand for this information. Food advisory label statements include the words "contains," "processed in a facility that also processes," and "may contain." Examples of food advisory labels might be as follows: Contains: milk, wheat, eggs (a listing of any of the top eight food allergens that are in the ingredients); Processed in a facility that also processes tree nuts (specific allergens); and May contain eggs (a specific allergen or allergens). If a food is labeled in this way, cross contamination is a strong possibility and best avoided by those with food allergies, intolerances, or sensitivities. In general, there is little risk for contamination with allergens in fresh vegetables, fruits, red meat, poultry, fish, pork, other meat products, and oils as long as they are not processed with other ingredients, exposed to allergenic food, or manufactured in a facility that processes food allergens.

In the United States studies show that the possibility for food allergy reactions remains even if a food label indicates no allergens because food labels often fail to accurately list ingredients. A study of food manufacturers in Minnesota, which was completed in 2000 by the U.S. Food and Drug Administration, found that approximately 25 percent of food manufacturers improperly labeled their food products or accidentally cross-contaminated food processed in their facilities.

It is always advisable to call food manufacturers to ask about their ingredients and manufacturing practices before eating a food that is not clearly labeled as allergen free. All food labels are required to provide telephone number of the manufacturer for consumer questions. It is also necessary to always recheck labels, because food manufacturers frequently change their ingredients and are not required to notify consumers about the change. It is also a good idea to visit the U.S. Food and Drug Administration website for food manufacturer violations. This federal agency lists food companies that have received warning letters or fines for food safety or labeling violations.

In general avoid buying foods in bulk food bins; deli meats and cheese; nut butters; baked goods, such as donuts, muffins, and pastries; and candy bars, baking pieces, baking chocolate, and other candies because cross-contamination risk is high.

Do not place safe and unsafe foods together in shopping carts unless allergen-free foods are put into a plastic bag before placement in the shopping cart to help prevent potential cross contamination.

26. Do food allergies, intolerances, and sensitivities have an impact on the emotional health of the individual and their family?

Food-sensitive individuals frequently become fearful, anxious, or stressed about having an adverse reaction to eating food. Children and adults may eat only specific foods every day, avoiding all new foods introduced into their diet. Or they may lose interest in eating or become depressed. Family members may also experience guilt for "giving" their family member a food allergy, become sad, eat out or travel infrequently, decrease social activities, or feel frustration about keeping them safe.

Many individuals with food allergies struggle with anxiety. It is important to have some anxiety, but excessive anxiety can be debilitating. A healthy anxiety reaction is to read food ingredient labels or question restaurant staff about meal preparation before eating any food. But for some people, the experience of having a food allergy reaction can result in excessive anxiety or post-traumatic stress reactions. Signs that an individual is suffering from an unhealthy anxiety response to his or her food allergy include fear of eating or severely limiting foods that are eaten in the daily diet, constant state of anxiousness, loss of sleep, and checking food ingredients over and over again, even after verifying they are safe to eat. The individual may also be afraid to eat out in restaurants, at a social function, or at a family or friend's home. Family caregivers may isolate allergic individuals to a separate room to eat away from the family to keep them safe.

Exploring these feelings of anxiety with a health-care professional specializing in this area can help the individual to better cope with fear and plan strategies to reduce the psychological toll food allergy reactions can have. For example, Dr. Scott Sicherer performs a touch test on kids with peanut butter allergies. He has his patients sniff peanut butter for 10 minutes and then apply a pea-sized amount of peanut butter on their skin for 1 minute. Very few of his patients have any type of adverse reaction, and those who do usually experience a minor reaction, such as red or itchy skin, or an anxiety reaction. Dr. Sicherer's touch test helps his patients to understand and experience that they can be around peanut butter and not have a reaction unless they eat it.

It is also helpful to explain that anxiety reactions can mimic food allergy reactions. Anxiety symptoms usually include hyperventilation, light headedness, muscle cramps, tingling, numb fingers, and difficulty breathing. These symptoms can be mistaken for a food allergy reaction. Education about these symptoms can ease anxiety and help the individual to distinguish between a real food allergy reaction and symptoms of anxiety. For children, the reassurance by parents and caregivers that the safety of their food is monitored often reduces anxiety. For adults, counselors, allergists, and trusted friends may be necessary to help them to reduce their feelings of anxiety related to eating.

27. Are there support groups available for individuals with food allergies, sensitivities, or intolerances?

There are many support groups available for those who struggle with food reactions.

Most food allergy research and education organizations offer local support groups.

Food Allergy Research & Education (FARE), Asthma and Allergy Foundation of America, No Nuts Moms, Food Allergy & Anaphylaxis Connection Team, and Kids with Food Allergies are some of the most well-known groups that organize local meetings, online chat groups, and virtual support groups. Allergists, gastroenterologists, and community public health departments may also be able to recommend support groups that are helpful and reliable.

It is important for anyone looking for a support group to research what services the group offers and their mission to ensure it is the right group for the individual.

Some things to consider and ask about before joining a support group include the following: Will a person's information be kept private and confidential? Are group times, activities, and location convenient and meet the individual's specific needs? Is the information provided by the group accurate and what are their information sources? Does a board-certified allergist support the group and does it have medical advisors? And are there any fees for joining the group and how are they used?

28. What resources are available to individuals with food allergies, sensitivities, and intolerances that can help them manage their daily life and meals more easily?

Food allergy organizations and peer groups often provide the most accurate and useful information to those who must manage food allergies, intolerances, and sensitivities. An individual's allergist or gastroenterologist and registered dietitian may also offer support and materials in their offices or hospitals where they practice.

The most reliable sources for information about every aspect of life when living with food reactions are the following organizations: Food Allergy Research & Education, Asthma & Allergy Foundation of America, and Food Allergy & Anaphylaxis Connection Team. Kids with Food Allergies is another reputable resource and a division of the Asthma & Allergy Foundation of America. In the United Kingdom, the Anaphylaxis Campaign provides many different resources for those with food allergies.

The Celiac Disease Foundation and the Crohn's & Colitis Foundation provide trustworthy resources helpful for those managing gastrointestinal-related intolerances and sensitivities. Other reputable resources include the Consortium of Food Allergy Research, National Institute of Allergy and Infectious Diseases, the FDA's Center for Food Safety and Applied Nutrition, Centers for Disease Control, FPIES Foundation, the International Association for Food Protein Entercolitis, American Partnership for Eosinophilic Disorders, Inflammatory Skin Disease Institute, Coalition of Skin Diseases, Jaffe Food Allergy Institute at Mount Sinai, American Academy of Allergy, Asthma, Immunology, Academy of Nutrition and Dietetics, American Academy of Pediatrics, and Food Allergy Canada.

Often family members of food allergy patients or patients themselves will start their own groups and websites, such as the No Nuts Moms group, Lactose Intolerance Global Network, and Irritable Bowel Syndrome Group. Various medical or naturopathic practices also offer information on their websites that may be helpful. However, information may not always be accurate on these websites, so it is essential to always learn more about these groups and where they get their information from.

The Past and Future: Food Allergy History, Current Research, and New Possibilities

29. How were food allergies first discovered?

Hippocrates, a Greek physician who is considered the "Father of Medicine" and practiced medicine from 460 BC to 370 BC, was the first physician to recognize that foods could affect health and well-being. According to "The Genuine Works of Hippocrates" by Francis Adams, Hippocrates wrote,

> For cheese does not prove equally injurious to all men, for there are some who can take it to satiety, without being hurt by it in the least, but, on the contrary, it is wonderful what strength it imparts to those it agrees with; but there are some who do not bear it well, their constitutions are different, they differ in this respect, that what in their body is incompatible with cheese, is roused and put in commotion by such a thing; and those in whose bodies such a humor happens to prevail in greater quantity and intensity, are likely to suffer the more from it. But if the thing had been pernicious to the whole nature of man, it would have hurt all.

Anaphylactic reactions have been recorded since the time of the ancient Egyptians. Hieroglyphics record the death of Pharaoh Menes from a wasp sting. But to understand the discovery of food allergies it is necessary to understand how the medical community discovered the immune system. The concept of immunity is first mentioned in the historical records of 5th-century Greece and 10th-century China. It was noted that people who survived common plagues during this time period were immune to them thereafter. Both Greece and China subsequently record using the technique of variolation to protect others from deadly plaques. Variolation exposed healthy people to a deadly disease, such as smallpox, by implanting infected lesion material caused by the disease under the skin or inhaling it through the nose. Often the patient would develop a mild case of the disease and a resulting immunity against it, thus increasing the chance for survival during an epidemic. However, since this method did not provide a standard amount of the virus, and could be stronger or weaker depending on the source material, some people did experience death or disfigurement from the technique.

During the 18th century, it was estimated that individuals had a 20–60 percent chance of death from smallpox. Smallpox is a painful disease that causes blisters both externally and internally. Survivors were often left scarred and sometimes blind. The worst strain of small pox is known as black pox, which causes hemorrhaging of blood. Smallpox was greatly feared, and the early concept of vaccination was developed to combat this disease. During the 1700s, Lady Mary Wortley Montagu introduced variolation to European countries. Cotton Mather introduced variolation to America in the 1700s, and the technique was employed during the Boston smallpox epidemic in 1721. In 1796, an English physician, Dr. Edward Jenner (1749–1823), noticed that milkmaids did not become ill with smallpox if they had been exposed to cowpox, a virus contracted from physical contact with cow udders during the milking process. Cowpox would cause a mild case of smallpox symptoms. In the first test to attempt protection against smallpox, Dr. Jenner took a cowpox scab and injected the pus into an eight-year-old boy, who was successfully protected against subsequent smallpox infections. Dr. Jenner published the results of his experiments in the *Inquiry into the Causes and Effects of the Variolae Vaccine* (1798). After Dr. Jenner's successful experiment, variolation was accepted by the medical community of the day and applied as a preventative measure against smallpox infection. Because the fear of smallpox was so great, by 1821 many countries made smallpox variolation of infants mandatory. It was soon discovered, however, that a one-time vaccination did not confer lifelong immunity. Infection rates were also high, since sterilized medical implements were not used at that time to give the injection often resulting in the loss of arm function or amputation. Unsterilized implements also spread diseases, such as leprosy and syphilis.

As societies evolved, the spread of infectious diseases became a major concern. Agrarian towns and villages were surrounded by farms and were more likely to have their drinking water contaminated with human and animal fecal matter, causing an increase in parasites and infections. Hunter and gather societies, such as the Incas and Aztec people, did not farm and raise animals and subsequently were not plagued with diseases as the agrarian societies were. As these agrarian societies changed over time, citizens began to move from rural areas and congregate in cities for jobs. Densely populated cities increased the likelihood and spread of disease, mainly due to improper sanitation practices. As society continued to evolve from hunter gather to agrarian to industrialized, city public health departments were formed to improve sanitation and deal with disease outbreaks. This in turn led to relying on vaccines to prevent fatal mass outbreaks of deadly diseases in densely populated areas.

The late 1800s also marked the beginning of fully understanding how diseases were transmitted from person to person. Up to this time, hygiene and sterile techniques were rarely used. But Dr. Joseph Lister (1827–1912), Dr. Robert Koch (1843–1910), and Dr. Louis Pasteur (1822–1895) validated the germ theory of disease, which is the idea that small microscopic organisms can cause disease and be spread from person to person. Sanitation also became recognized as important in the prevention of disease. Dr. Ignaz Semmelweis (1818–1865) attempted to educate his colleagues about washing hands before attending to women during childbirth to prevent the death of the mother, which was at epidemic levels at that time. In 1854, public health worker John Snow convinced London officials that a communal well contaminated with feces was the source of an outbreak of cholera.

Dr. Pasteur, considered the father of immunology, found that weakened strains of bacteria could confer immunity, and this discovery, along with the new hypodermic needle, marked the beginning of modern-day vaccination techniques. The early 1900s saw rapid discoveries of biomedical and immunology science and clinical practice developments. Mass vaccination programs became an accepted practice to prevent disease among the population. The ingredients added to vaccines also evolved quickly to make them as safe as possible, reduce serum sickness, and increase their shelf life. Serum sickness was a common reaction at that time that resulted from injections of antiserum and is similar to vaccine reactions today. But reactions to vaccination could not be eliminated completely. Because public health officials felt the benefits of vaccines outweighed the risks, and also to protect vaccine manufacturers financially, governments protected vaccine manufacturers from disclosing vaccine ingredients and from lawsuits. As medicines and vaccines evolved, the first modern-day pharmaceutical company, Parke-Davis, was established in 1866. The current model of allergy research subsequently evolved from the study of mass vaccine injuries. Forced vaccinations by many governments was common during this time but came into question by many doctors and mothers, who resisted. This topic is explored in George Bernard Shaw's 1909 book *The Doctor's Dilemma.*

French physiologist Francois Magendie (1783–1855) discovered that animals sensitized to egg white via injections experienced anaphylaxis and death when injected with them a second time. While individuals did experience anaphylactic reactions, it was not until the beginning of the 20th century that these reactions began to occur with increased frequency among children. It was during this time that the hypodermic syringe was first used to administer antitoxin sera in the new technique of vaccination. Serum sickness or death occurred frequently after the introduction of the hypodermic syringe method of vaccination, and parents often had to choose between the fear of an adverse reaction to a vaccine and the consequences of a deadly infectious disease. Charles Richet (1850–1935) and Dr. Clemens von Pirquet (1874–1929) subsequently showed in their research studies that vaccine injections lead to the first allergy epidemic in children.

Immunologist Dr. Charles Richet coined the term "anaphylaxis" ("ana" meaning "against" and "phylaxis" meaning "protection") after injecting dogs with toxins to protect them against future exposures. Dogs that survived the initial dose of toxins were given a second shot and expected to be protected against the toxin. However, the dogs became violently ill and died, indicating that they had developed a hypersensitivity to the toxin. The reaction depended on the amount of time between injections and not on the dose. Richet noted in his acceptance speech for the 1913 Nobel Prize in medicine that there were three possible outcomes of vaccination: unchanged sensitivity or stability, diminished sensitivity or habituation, and heightened sensitivity. He stated: "The first injection, instead of protecting the organism rendered it more fragile and susceptible" (Richet, 1913). Research by Nicolas Arthus (1862–1945) in 1903 and Richard Otto in 1905 confirmed that all proteins considered toxic or nontoxic outside the body could produce anaphylaxis without exception.

Throughout history physicians have altered a patient's diet when treating illness. The first physician to spend significant time treating negative food reactions was Dr. Francis Hare of Brisbane, Australia. His 1905 book, *The Food Factor in Disease*, reviewed his experience with foods that caused migraine headaches in his patients. His treatment for migraines included restricting fats, carbohydrates, and alcoholic beverages. He also diagnosed asthma, biliousness, bronchitis, dyspepsia, eczema, epilepsy, gout, headache, hypertension, mania, migraine, nervousness, and other degenerative diseases common in his day to be connected with food allergies.

In 1906 an Austrian pediatrician, Dr. Clemens von Pirquet, was the first medical professional to use the term "allergy." He suggested that any form of altered biological reactivity, such as a hypersensitivity resulting in tissue damage, should be classified as an allergy. Those who experienced a reaction to mosquito or bee stings, had hay fever, or had serum sickness were classified as having an allergy. Dr. von Pirquet also termed food allergy as an inappropriate reaction to food or other substances not typically harmful. Richet discovered through experiments with dogs, cats, rabbits, horse, and frogs that the body's response to food proteins introduced via the bloodstream without the process of digestion sensitized the animals, making them more susceptible to hypersensitivity reactions. However, most of Dr. von Pirquet's medical colleagues rejected his classification of allergies and refused to accept that immunity could work against the body for a number of years.

In the meantime in England in 1908, Dr. Alfred Schofield (1846–1929) reported successfully treating a boy with angioedema and asthma by restricting eggs in the boy's diet. *The Journal of Urology* in 1917 published an article written by Drs. W. T. Longcope and M. Rachemann that documented six patients with urticaria and renal insufficiency symptoms that were caused by negative food reactions. Dr. W. W. Duke also published an article in *The Archives of Internal Medicine*, *Journal of the American Medical Association*, and *Annals of Clinical Medicine* (1921, 1923) reporting food-related medical illnesses.

But food allergy reactions were still not much of a concern in the public or medical community until the 1930s, when a small number of people began to experience anaphylaxis after consuming cottonseed oil. The FDA, after performing an investigation into the matter, concluded that poor cottonseed manufacturing production methods had allowed the oil to become contaminated. But this discovery did not determine exactly why people were experiencing allergic reactions since cottonseed oil had been regularly consumed without incident prior to this. Cottonseed oil allergic reactions continued until the 1950s, when they began to decline and become rare. This decline coincides with the removal of cottonseed oil used in foods and medications, but a more thorough investigation into the cause at that time was never completed.

Food allergy research began to advance in 1931 when Dr. Albert Rowe published his study results in *Food Allergy: Its Manifestations, Diagnosis, and Treatment*. In 1972 he and his son published updates in *Food Allergy: Its Manifestations and Control and Elimination Diets—A Compendium*. In 1941, Dr. Warren Vaughan, an allergist, published his book *Strange Malady* in which he concluded that peanuts were not much of an allergy concern at that time. In his clinical practice he saw allergies most commonly to milk, egg, corn, soybean, cottonseed, shrimp, tomato, cabbage, cherry, chocolate, strawberries, and other foods. But rarely did he encounter a peanut allergy. But by 1948 peanut sensitivity became an emerging concern after penicillin vaccines that contained a peanut oil additive were given to children. Dr. Theron G. Randolph (1906–1995), an American allergist who practiced during the 1950s and 1960s, became increasingly convinced that many illnesses were caused by sensitivities and allergy reactions to foods and environmental inhalants and chemicals. By 1956 increased attention was turned to peanut allergy reactions due to an increase in reactions to peanuts.

In the 1960s, in an effort to more precisely distinguish between types of allergy reactions, British immunologists P.G.H. Gell (1914–2001) and R.R.A. Coombs (1921–2006) described four types of hypersensitivity reactions: anaphylactic, cytolytic, inflammatory, and cellular. Anaphylactic reactions involved immediate release of pharmacological active substances, like histamine, that triggered a response from the immune system. Cytolytic reactions involved antigens and antibodies that worked together to destroy cells. Inflammatory reactions produced excess antigens or antibodies in the body. Cellular reactions were initiated by white blood cells of the immune system and not antibodies.

Still, food allergy reactions were not considered a real medical illness until the mid-1970s when Dr. Charles May and Dr. Allan Bock defined the biological aspect of food allergies and established the use of double-blind, placebo-controlled oral food challenges as a diagnostic procedure for food allergy diagnosis. Because of the objectivity of this testing method, food allergy research began to be taken seriously by the medical community. In 1973, the first U.S. study of peanut allergy was conducted. By the 1980s medical researchers identified the proteins in peanuts that triggered an allergic reaction, Ara h 1 and Ara h 2. Austrian physician Hans Seyle (1907–1982) studied the physical response to stress and its connection to chronic illness and sensitivities. Dr. Seyle suggested that many clinical conditions, including allergy, rheumatoid arthritis, and hypertension, were "manifestations of the body's adaptive reactions, its mechanism of defense against stress" (Jackson, 2006, p. 203). Dr. Seyle identified three phases of a "general adaption syndrome" to neurological, immunological, and endocrinological stress response. These were the alarm phase, the stage of resistance or adaptation, and the stage of exhaustion. During the alarm phase, the body reacts immediately to combat the stressor. This would include hay fever, asthma, and anaphylactic shock due to exposure to a food allergen or environmental toxin. During the resistance or adaptation stage, the body works to maintain homeostasis despite constant exposure to a stressor. This would involve masking the cause for the reaction by the body. The state of exhaustion is the point when the body can no longer maintain its equilibrium, leading to multiple sensitivities or death.

The death of 10-year-old Boston native Michael Grzybinski in 1972 and an 18-year-old Brown University student in 1986 lead to the increasing and strong public outcry for robust and transparent food allergy labeling laws. As food allergies began to be considered a real medical concern, the public began to raise many concerns about the food supply that continues today. By the 1980s, food manufacturer Nestlé became actively involved in allergy research and formulated a partially hydrolyzed milk formula for babies allergic to milk. This altered formula reduced mast cell (IgE) response and thus allergic reactions. By the 1990s, a dramatic increase in peanut allergy anaphylactic reactions and deaths was seen. Clinicians began to rapidly strive to raise awareness, encourage patients to wear medical alert bracelets, and called for the food industry to clearly label food products with allergy warnings. Many governments and countries began to legislate regulations enforcing clear labeling laws, and increased efforts were put into food allergy research. Ongoing research continues today into the root cause of food allergy reactions.

30. How were food sensitivities and food intolerances first distinguished from food allergies?

It is difficult to pinpoint exactly when food sensitivities and intolerances were distinguished from "true" food allergies because sensitivities and intolerances are usually lumped together in the allergy category. But for centuries doctors recognized that people react differently to food. Food intolerances and sensitivities, which are responsible for an estimated 95 percent of food reactions, are only just recently becoming recognized as valid medical reactions as the nature of food allergy is better understood and knowledge increases about gastrointestinal system involvement with immunity and health.

Some food intolerances have been known for centuries. Dr. Fabrizio Bartoletti (1576–1630) discovered lactose in 1619. There was little evidence of lactose intolerance among world populations, except in those who were born without the gene that makes lactase enzyme. It is surmised that lactose intolerance was first seen due to a genetic variation that occurred about 8,000 years ago when humans started milking domesticated cows, goats, and sheep. Galactosemia was discovered in 1908 and recognized as a medical condition in 1917. Fructose was discovered in 1794, but fructose intolerance and malabsorption were not recognized as medical disorders until the 1960s.

The 1960s saw the emergence of environmental concerns related to health. Rachel Carson's *Silent Spring* in 1962 brought public awareness to the forefront as more evidence became known about the effects on health from pesticide use on foods. This increased awareness started an environmental movement in the 1970s that focused on how crops were grown and animals fed and nurtured to adulthood. Dr. Theron G. Randolph and Dr. Richard Mackarness (1916–1996), both environmental allergists, alerted the public to the rising trend of allergies due to chemical adulteration of foods. Dr. Randolph described food reactions as "the interaction between you and your own particular environment, which is different from anyone else's" (Ibid., 2006, p. 208). Clinical ecologists championed this area in direct conflict with the medical community, who felt these theories were unsubstantiated and led to the Royal College of Physicians 2003 statement that "food allergy is the cause of much controversy" (Royal College of Physicians, 2003, p. 52). The Royal College of Physicians concluded that "food intolerance is a more difficult and poorly defined area, where there is much less evidence on which to base practice" (Ibid., p. 56). Lack of objective evidence led many conventional practitioners to conclude that many patients with food intolerance had an underlying mental illness rather than an immunological disorder.

Around 8000 BCE, wheat was cultivated and used for food. Modern-day wheat composition has changed from its original composition due to cross-breeding crop techniques and the use of genetically modified seeds. This altered composition is theorized to cause intolerances and sensitivities since some people are unable to digest this new wheat because the gastrointestinal system has not evolved in the way it digests foods. Dr. Willem Dicke (1905–1962) discovered celiac disease in the 1940s and used a wheat-free diet to successfully treat patients. In 1944 the Netherlands experienced a famine, which improved the health of celiac patients and confirmed a wheat-free diet as a treatment method. But diagnostic methods for gluten intolerance did not come into existence until 1956. Non-celiac gluten sensitivities were recognized in 2012 by celiac researchers and differentiated as a valid medical condition.

The majority of food intolerances and sensitivities have only been recently recognized, and many still remain controversial. Dr. Benjamin Feingold (1900–1982), an American pediatrician, increased awareness about food additives and resulting health problems when he published his book *Why Your Child Is Hyperactive* (1974). Dr. Feingold was convinced that attention deficit hyperactivity disorder was linked with food additives. He prescribed the Feingold Diet, which removed all food additives in the diet, to his patients with some success. In the 1990s research focus shifted from food allergies to allergies and sensitivities to synthetic food preservatives and colorings. Biophysicist Richard Cone and anthropologist Emily Martin published a 1997 article in the *Ecologist*, "Corporeal Flows: The Immune System, Global Economies of Food, and Implications for Health," stating that humans were increasingly living in disharmony with their environment. The modern diet was implicated because most people were no longer consuming local produce, instead eating more processed foods and foods that were produced far away. This in turn limited their ability to come in contact with proteins that matched those in the body, leading to illness and chronic illnesses such as arthritis. Pesticides and preservatives exacerbated this problem by tricking the immune system into reacting to harmless food proteins as toxins. Dr. Alessio Fasano, a pediatric gastroenterologist and research scientist, is recognized for his research of celiac disease and gluten intolerance. In 2000, his research team discovered the molecule zonulin, which regulates the permeability of the intestine. It was subsequently found that increased zonulin levels were prominent in those with celiac disease and leaky gut, even after gluten was removed from the diet. However, traditional gastroenterologists do not yet believe there is adequate evidence to support the diagnosis of leaky gut syndrome. Food sensitivities require much more research and remain controversial within the medical community.

31. What is the history of diagnosis methods for food allergies, intolerances, and sensitivities?

Food allergy diagnostic tests used today include the skin prick test, IgE antibody blood testing, oral food challenge, and trial elimination diet. But the first test used to diagnose food allergy was the patch test in 1896 by a German dermatologist, Dr. Josef Jadasshon (1853–1936). The patch test involved applying a patch with the trigger substance on the skin and monitoring the skin for changes. In 1908, injections under the skin of trigger substances were used instead of patches to ellicit allergy reactions. American pediatrician Oscar Menderson Schloss (1882–1952) was the first pediatrician to diagnose food allergies using the skin prick test in 1912. Research by Carl Pausnitz (1876–1963) and Heinz Küstner (1897–1963) in 1912 showed that reactivity to a substance could be transferred to the blood. Dr. Küstner, who was allergic to cooked fish, experienced an immediate and positive skin test response after eating cooked fish. This blood serum transfer of reactivity to the skin was termed the "P-K response." Extensively researched by Helmtraud Erbuster, the skin prick test became the primary diagnostic tool for type I hypersensitivity reactions by 1959.

In 1900, Paul Ehrlich (1854–1915), who is considered one of the fathers of immunology, hypothesized that there was an antibody molecule that linked with an antigen. In 1906, pediatrician Clemens von Pirquet identified the term "supersensitivity without immunity" to describe symptoms of inhaled allergy and immediate skin reactions to a substance when immunity tests were negative.

Clemens von Pirquet devised a test for reactions to tuberculin, an antigen used in tuberculosis inoculation by 1907. Dr. Chandler Walker (1883–1950) further developed von Pirquet's test to identify most allergens using skin prick or scratch tests. But the dangers of a severe reaction to the test and the high percentage of inaccurate test results led many allergists, including Drs. Rowe, Rinkel, and Randolph, to conclude most skin tests at the time were unreliable diagnostic methods. Because of this, the elimination diet was formulated by Dr. Albert Rowe and initially called the Rowe diet. Rowe introduced the food elimination diet in 1929, later publishing *Elimination Diets and the Patient's Allergies*. He believed that every food could trigger allergy reactions and that food allergens remained in the blood for long periods of time. His diet was very restrictive and had to be followed over a long period of time. Medical professionals questioned the nutritional adequacy of his diet, especially when used with children. But his elimination diet became accepted practice in many allergy offices by the 1930s. His diet was revised over the decades because patients had a difficult time adhering to it. In the early 1920s, Herbert Rinkel refined the skin prick tests, using a five-fold serial dilution of food extract that was adjusted to a patient's sensitivity that was administered just under the skin. Known at the Rinkel method, it too had a number of inaccurate results. Many allergists of the day used a combination of the Rinkel method and elimination diet to confirm an allergy diagnosis.

By 1935, R. A. Cooke identified that antibodies in the blood increased during sensitivity reactions, and in 1934, Warren Vaughan identified two types of white blood cells that were elevated in food reactions. Vaughn developed the leukopenic index, which measured leucocytes in the blood before and three times after a meal was eaten. This method was controversial since exercise, emotion, and timing of the meal could elevate leucocytes as well. In 1948, Astrid Fagraeus (1913–1997) discovered that B cells were specifically involved in antibody production. In 1940, Linus Pauling (1901–1994) proposed that antigens acted as a template for an antibody, but in 1957 Frank Burnet and David Talmage determined that lymphocytes produced single specific antibody molecules. Dr. Arthur Coca devised the Coca pulse test in the 1950s. Dr. Coca developed this test after his wife reported her pulse "raced" after eating certain foods. Many clinicians were skeptical of this test and did not consider an accurate method of diagnosis.

By 1966, the IgE antibody was identified as a reliable indicator of an allergy reaction, and Gerald Edelman and Rodney Porter identified the molecular structure of antibodies. In 1967 the radioallergosorbent test (RAST) was developed as a diagnostic test to detect allergen antibodies. The year 1975 marked the beginning of modern-day antibody research that continues today. Dr. Charles May introduced the oral food challenge test in the mid-1970s. Until this time many medical professionals were skeptical that food allergies were a valid medical condition. But use of the double-blind, placebo-controlled oral food challenge provided an evidence-based method to validate the food allergy reaction. By 1978 elimination diets were accepted as a useful and valid diagnostic tool by the medical community. The radioactive isotope used to identify antibodies in the RAST was replaced in 1989 with enzymatic substances, and the test is now called ImmunoCAP.

The 1970s through the 2000s also marked the beginning of alternative testing methods for food reactions discussed in Question 7, such as muscle testing, cytotoxicity testing, electrodermal tests, natural elimination of allergy treatment and Nambrudipad's allergy elimination technique, IgG and IgG4 testing, hair analysis, hydrogen breath tests, and pulse testing. Cytotoxicity testing, also called Bryan's Test, dated back to 1947. The ALCAT test originated in 1988. All of these methods remain controversial as valid diagnostic tests today.

32. What is currently being done to improve food allergy testing and diagnosis methods?

Traditional testing methods focus on IgE antibody detection. While IgE tests have been the most extensively researched, there is ongoing and active research about non-IgE- and IgE-associated reactions and diseases. The goal of improved diagnostic methods is to increase accuracy and identify severity and prognosis of food allergies.

One new testing method that is approved for use in Europe and for peanut allergy in the United States is component testing. Currently allergy testing separates and tests individual food proteins. Component testing evaluates a collection of pure allergen food proteins rather than individual allergen protein extracts because they represent a mixture of allergenic and nonallergenic components that more closely mimic food. The theory of component testing is that foods contain many allergens, and component testing increases the ability to determine which protein is actually causing a reaction. For example, it is known that the peanut protein Ara h 2 is difficult to digest and associated with severe reactions. Ara h 8 is easy to digest and associated with either no peanut allergy reaction or a mild one. But a person can be allergic to either one or both. Current testing cannot distinguish which of the proteins is causing the reaction. But component testing evaluates both proteins together to accurately identify which protein fraction elicits the allergic reaction. While component testing shows promise, only the peanut allergen component test has been approved for use in the United States. Research is still needed, however, to determine if component testing is reliable when evaluating other food allergens. Component testing for all allergens is used in Europe however. While this newer testing method appears more accurate, it still does not replace traditional diagnostic test and oral food challenges and is used as one more tool to accurately diagnose food allergies. A 2013 *Current Allergy & Asthma Reports* article discusses allergen component testing in depth.

Another new test method that looks promising is in vitro food allergy diagnosis using immunoassays and aptamer-based assays, including immunoaffinity capillary electrophoresis. Aptamers are single-strand DNA or RNA oligonucleotides with a specific sequence that attracts a particular target molecule, such as a food allergen. Immunological assays detect a specific food molecule by using magnetic nanoparticles. These methods provide a more accurate and rapid identification method of food allergens present in the blood, appearing to improve the accuracy of food allergy diagnosis. But use as a diagnostic tool still requires more research.

Epitope testing is another diagnostic method that shows promise. Every food protein has various identifying areas on its molecular structure that can be recognized by the immune system. Those specific locations are thought to affect how a person reacts to them and may possibly be connected to an allergic response. However, research is only just beginning into epitope testing as a useful diagnostic tool.

Affinity testing is a new method that evaluates the strength of IgE attachment to a protein. It is speculated that the stronger this attachment, the more severe or persistent an allergy will be. But research into this theory is only just beginning, and no indication of its usefulness as a diagnostic tool is yet available. Research into other areas is ongoing.

33. What is current research discovering about food allergies, intolerances, and sensitivities?

While past research has limitations in its application mostly due to study design that can lead to biased results, many studies that are specifically designed to eliminate bias toward the results are currently in progress. Research studies usually belong in two categories. One category is conducted in a lab setting with animals. The other category involves research that studies people. There are two types of research methods used to study a subject. One type evaluates a specific subject, and the other focuses on finding therapies that will work in the treatment of that subject. Most study funding comes from federal governments using tax dollars. But some are funded through private corporations and donors. All research studies are regulated and supervised to ensure animal or participant safety and adequate study design. Review committees analyze study design, methods, and conclusions to ensure valid results.

When study theories are validated by other studies, the proposed research subject advances to clinical trials. Clinical trials are studies that evaluate a therapy or treatment for safety and effectiveness with humans. There are five phases of a clinical trial: Phase 0, Phase I, Phase II, Phase III, and Phase IV. Each phase builds on the previous phase and is specifically designed to answer predetermined conclusions. For example, when new pharmaceutical drugs are developed, Phase 0 studies are exploratory studies that use only small doses of the new drug in a small number of patients to minimize risk. Phase I studies include more study subjects and have the goal of finding the highest dose of a new treatment that can be given safely without serious side effects. This phase has the most risk associated with it. The clinical trial will then progress to Phase II only if

Phase I results are reasonably safe. Phase II studies usually include more people than Phase I. If side effects are minimal, the trial will then progress to Phase III. Phase III trials have the largest number of patients, are often done in more than one country, and tend to last longer than the other phases. The goal of Phase III trials is to prove safety of a new treatment before approving it for general use in patients. If a treatment is safe and effective, if it is a drug, the manufacturer will then submit a new drug application to the appropriate government regulatory agency before the drug is used in medical practice. Phase IV studies have also been used to evaluate drugs that have been on the market for a long period of time. The goal of the Phase IV study is to evaluate long-term safety of a treatment.

Most research done to date has been about IgE allergy reactions. The only treatment for these allergies is strict avoidance of the trigger food. But one new treatment method that has met with some success involves injecting a trigger protein that binds and inactivates IgE into a person. The theory of this treatment method is that inactivating the body's response of IgE will prevent an allergic reaction. This treatment method has been effective in individuals with chronic allergic asthma that has not responded well to other therapies. But more research is still needed to ensure safety in larger populations. Allergy shots have also been used for a number of years for individuals with pollen allergies. Allergy shots are immunotherapy injections of proteins that cause pollen and insect allergies. They have been protective against a reaction, and they are thought to reeducate the immune system to not attack the injected proteins. Studies in the 1980s injected participants with peanut proteins, but reactions were severe, and this treatment method for peanut allergy was abandoned. So far, allergy shots have not been successful in the treatment of food allergies.

The most promising new allergen treatment methods for non-IgE allergies include desensitization to trigger foods. Desensitization means that an individual is able to consume a trigger food without experiencing a reaction. It is thought it may be an effective method of protection against potentially fatal reactions because desensitization protection is not permanent in the long term. Research continues into this promising area.

Immunotherapies are also being researched as one way for a person to develop protective immunological changes that may protect against a reaction. These therapies include oral immunotherapy and sublingual immunotherapy. Oral immunotherapy involves exposing a patient to small but steadily increased doses of a food allergen until the person becomes desensitized to it. The Food Allergy Research & Education group (FARE) has completed much research in this area, and it has concluded that this is a safe and promising treatment for food allergy. FARE clinical studies to date find that 50–70 percent of patients given oral immunotherapy experience a complete desensitization to the trigger food being studied. However, adverse reactions were still frequent with common symptoms of abdominal pain, wheezing, and diarrhea. Although oral immunotherapy is still not considered to be a safe treatment for IgE-mediated allergies, oral immunotherapy does show promise as an effective treatment for non-IgE-mediated food reactions. More studies regarding safety and efficacy are needed in this research area.

FARE founded Aimmune Therapeutics, Inc., to study oral immunotherapy in depth. Currently Aimmune Therapeutics is researching clinical trials for peanut allergy and egg allergy. Aimmune Therapeutics developed a treatment called AR101. AR101 is a defatted, lightly roasted peanut flour containing the most common peanut antigens. AR101 powder is used as an oral immunotherapy to support the desensitization of an individual to peanut proteins. Aimmune Therapeutics is currently conducting Phase III clinical trials using AR101, including the Peanut Allergy Oral Immunotherapy Study of AR101 for Desensitization in Children and Adults (PALISADE), the Real World AR101 Market Supporting Experience Study in peanut allergic children (RAMSES), and the AR101 Trial in Europe Measuring Oral Immunotherapy Success (ARTEMIS) studies. The PALISADE clinical trial enrolled over 550 participants aged 4–55 from the United States, Canada, and Europe with the goal to evaluate the efficacy and safety of AR101 to treat peanut allergy. The RAMSES study began enrolling participants aged 4–17 in the United States and Canada in May 2017. The goal of the RAMSES study is to evaluate the desensitization to peanuts in a real-world setting without the use of a food challenge. The ARTEMIS clinical trial also began enrolling participants aged 4–17 in Europe in July 2017. The goal of ARTEMIS is to study the length of time it takes for these participants to become desensitized to peanuts. While it will be sometime before study results are available, Phase II clinical trial results for AR101 were published in the March/April 2018 publication of *The Journal of Allergy and Clinical Immunology in Practice*. This study used a randomized, double-blind, placebo-controlled design that desensitized eligible participants aged 4–26 years to peanuts. Fifty-five patients were randomized into groups that received either AR101 or a placebo. Results showed AR101 safety was acceptable, and AR101 demonstrated an effective immunomodulatory treatment for young children, adolescents, and young adults.

Sublingual immunotherapy uses a technique that dissolves a food allergen in a solution, and small drops of this allergen extract are then administered to patients under their tongue. Small doses are started and then increased as tolerated. Some sublingual immunotherapy studies show they are effective in preventing asthma and allergic rhinoconjuctivitis. Studies using it for kiwi, hazelnut, milk, peach, and peanut allergies showed promising results of its use as an effective treatment. D. M. Fleischer and his colleagues published the results of a randomized, double-blind, placebo-controlled multicenter trial of sublingual therapy for peanut allergy in the *Journal of Allergy and Clinical Immunology* in 2013. Forty participants were enrolled in this study, and 70 percent were shown to become safely desensitized to peanuts. However, subsequent studies do find sublingual immunotherapy only minimally desensitizes a patient to a trigger food. Adverse reactions were also more common to sublingual immunotherapy than to oral immunotherapy. While not as effective as oral immunotherapy, it still shows promise in preventing potentially fatal reactions. Studies that combine oral immunotherapy and sublingual immunotherapy therapies also show promise. C. A. Keet and colleagues reported in the *Journal of Allergy and Clinical Immunology* in 2012 that 10 percent of sublingual immunotherapy, 60 percent of sublingual immunotherapy and oral immunotherapy of 1,000 mg of milk protein, and 80 percent of sublingual immunotherapy and oral immunotherapy of 2,000 mg of milk protein study participants were desensitized to milk protein. While all are promising, they are still not approved for food allergy treatment, and more safety and effectiveness trials are needed.

One other area of immunotherapy involves the use of epicutaneous immunotherapy. This treatment involves rubbing a trigger food on the skin for prolonged periods of time to allow absorption through the skin into the circulatory system. The theory for this therapy is that immune cells in the skin may desensitize a person to the food over time. This method is unlikely to trigger severe reactions, and early studies show that some patients are able to have increased amounts of a trigger food over time. A National Institutes of Health-funded study reported in 2016 that a wearable patch that delivered small amounts of peanut protein through the skin allowed participants to eat at least 10 times more peanut protein than prior to the study. Treatment was especially effective for younger children and was safely tolerated. Studies investigating its use with peanut and milk allergies are ongoing.

Chinese herbal therapies also show promise as effective treatments for food allergy as well. Data from mice studies reported in the 2012 issue of *Current Allergy Asthma Reports* found a Chinese herbal allergy formulation, composed of nine herbal extracts and called FAHF-2, protected against peanut allergic reactions when the mice were challenged with oral peanut foods. However, continued research into this treatment is needed regarding safety and effectiveness.

Probiotics, prebiotics, and synbiotics are also being tried as a food allergy treatment. Probiotics are live microorganisms that live in the gastrointestinal system and confer benefits when taken in adequate amounts. Prebiotics are nutrients that support healthy bacterial growth in the gastrointestinal tract.

Synbiotics are a combination of the two. *Frontiers in Pediatrics* published an informative article on allergy and asthma probiotic research in 2017. This article highlighted results that show preclinical studies find probiotics modify the gastrointestinal microbiome, subsequently reducing sensitization and allergic inflammation and possibly protecting the individual against asthma and allergic reactions. However, most study results to date show poor effectiveness when using probiotics for treating food allergies.

Using helminth parasites as an allergy treatment is also being explored. Treatment that uses the Trichuris suis ova (TSO) of the pig whipworm is currently being studied as an allergy treatment. TSO worms are given in capsule form, where they hatch in the intestine. The TSO parasite does not live long in humans, and treatment given for this parasite involves the same cells and proteins that the immune system uses during an allergic response. Several studies in animals find that using an intestinal helminth infection can inhibit the development of intestinal inflammation. Long-term studies find TSO treatment has been beneficial for ulcerative colitis and Crohn's patients. While promising, other studies find that TSO may not be as protective against an allergy reaction if allergic reactivity is already established. The thought behind TSO treatment is that having these parasites short term will promote less allergic response. However, this theory remains controversial since it may also increase the body's reactivity. Helminth infections can cause unintended illnesses as well.

Peanut vaccines are one other area that is currently being researched. Jessica O'Konek, lead researcher of a 2018 study investigating peanut vaccines, delivered a nano-emulsion vaccine in the form of a nasal spray of very fine peanut protein droplets combined with purified soybean oil, detergents, and water to peanut-sensitive mice. The mice in the study were protected against mild to more severe reactions to peanuts. Results are promising, and research continues in the area of food vaccines.

Case Studies

CASE STUDY 1

Jason is a 20-year-old freshman college student. He is excited about starting college but is also worried because he has a tree nut allergy. Diagnosed when he was 10 years old, Jason first experienced an anaphylactic reaction after eating trail mix that included tree nuts during a school-hiking trip. He had never had any reaction to eating tree nuts prior to this. Luckily his teachers were carrying EpiPens® with them and administered emergency treatment to Jason. He was transported to a hospital, where he was observed and stabilized. He was subsequently seen by his pediatrician and tested for food allergies. Jason's skin prick tests were inconclusive, but his blood tests showed an elevated IgE level to tree nuts only, indicating he had a tree nut allergy. His tree nut allergy was confirmed when he was given a double-blind, placebo-controlled food challenge. The test was performed in his local hospital to ensure his safety in the event he had a severe reaction. Jason experienced anaphylaxis during the test. Because of his age, the fact that he was still growing, and the possibility that he could develop nutrient deficiencies from eliminating tree nuts in his diet, his parents brought him to see a registered dietitian. The registered dietitian evaluated Jason and planned a nutritionally balanced and healthy diet plan for him that would help prevent any possible nutrient deficiencies and promoted appropriate growth for his age. She also educated Jason and his family about his eating plan, how to manage it, and strategies to help them and him safely manage his nut allergy. Jason and his family learned that reading food labels and questioning cooks, kitchen and waitstaff, and anyone who prepared food for him was the most important strategy that they could employ to avoid allergic reactions. Because anxiety is a common reaction among individuals with food allergies and their family members, his mother joined a local food allergy support group to help her cope with her anxiety and worry about Jason having a fatal allergy reaction.

Jason has always been very careful to eat foods he knows do not have tree nuts, and he always carries an EpiPen® with him at all times in case of an accidental reaction. Prior to Jason's first semester at his college, he notified the dining hall manager about his tree nut allergy. The dining staff at his college undergoes food allergy training every semester, learning how to recognize and respond to food allergy reactions. They also learn proper sanitation and food preparation procedures to avoid cross contamination of food with allergenic foods and how to prepare allergen-free snacks and meals. Jason feels confident that his meals in the dining hall are safe for him to eat. But picking nut-free snacks in the cafeteria has been more of a challenge for him. He usually buys nut-free snacks that he keeps in his dorm room. But today he ran out of his snacks and needs to carry some snacks with him because he has a long day filled with classes that will prevent him from eating a meal until late in the day. He must pick something from the dining hall and selects a granola bar from the cafeteria that, after reading the food label, appears to have no tree nuts in the ingredients. He has eaten this particular granola bar before and had no allergy reactions. But he double-checks with the cashier, who also thinks the granola bar will be safe. Jason eats half of the granola bar before he begins to feel light headed and then begins to have difficulty breathing. Luckily he is walking to class with his best friend, Steve, who recognizes Jason's symptoms. Steve digs through Jason's backpack and finds his EpiPen®. Steve administers a shot of epinephrine to Jason and then quickly calls 911 on his cell phone. Within five minutes emergency services arrive. Jason's ability to breathe began to improve after he received the epinephrine injection, but his face is beginning to swell. He is stabilized by the emergency responders and taken to the hospital for follow-up care and observation.

Analysis

Managing food allergies can sometimes be difficult, especially when a person must rely on prepackaged foods as Jason had to that day. This case highlights the need for an individual to always be vigilant, even if a trusted brand has been eaten before without incident. Question 7 reviewed the food allergy testing methods that were used to confirm Jason's tree nut allergy. Because he was young at the time of his diagnosis and still growing, it was possible that he could develop nutrient deficiencies from eliminating nuts from his diet as he grew. He and his family also needed to learn how to manage his food allergy so that he could live a normal life. As Question 23 discusses in depth, he was evaluated by a registered dietitian, who planned a nutritionally adequate diet for him that would ensure proper growth and avoid any possible nutrient deficiencies. His dietitian also taught Jason and his family how to successfully manage his tree nut allergy by educating them about food preparation and sanitation techniques, how to shop for prepared and processed foods in the supermarket, and how to eat away from home safely.

Because anxiety is a common reaction among individuals with food allergies and their family members, as explored in Questions 26 and 27, Jason's mother joined a local food allergy group to manage her worry about Jason possibly having a fatal reaction. Jason did not develop anxiety over his food allergy but did have a healthy concern about his safety and always made sure his friends and teachers knew what to do if he should have an allergy reaction. Emergency treatment for allergic reactions is detailed in Question 21. Because his good friend Steve had known Jason since they were three, Steve had seen Jason experience an allergy reaction before. Steve was very aware of the symptoms of a food allergy reaction and knew how to respond in case of an emergency. Steve was also aware of where to locate Jason's emergency care kit if needed.

But as Question 24 highlights, one of the most common mistakes individuals with a food allergy make is to assume a food is safe before eating it. In this case, the granola bar he selected was processed in a manufacturing facility that also processed tree nuts. As Questions 24 and 25 detail, the Food Allergen Labeling and Consumer Protection Act in the United States requires food manufacturers to list common major food allergens on their labels. However, they are not required to list whether a food is processed in a facility that also manufactures allergenic foods. Because of this, unless the food label specifically stated that it is manufactured in an allergen-free facility, there is an increased possibility that the granola bar Jason chose could have been accidentally contaminated with tree nuts. An investigation into the incident revealed that the production line used for the manufacturer of the granola bar had trace amounts of tree nuts. This indicated that the production line was not adequately cleansed between food products, leading to this cross-contamination incident. This food manufacturer had also been cited in the past for previous sanitation violations.

What could Jason have done to prevent or minimize his risk for an allergic reaction that day? One strategy is to always replenish his snack supply before he runs out so that his "safe" snacks are always available. But, in this case, he was unable to get to a supermarket to buy his snacks until the weekend. Another strategy he could have used was to speak with his dining hall manager about always having allergen-free snacks available in the dining hall when needed. Jason should also periodically call food manufacturers to confirm that no ingredients had been changed in the snacks he usually eats, and he should also visit the U.S. Food & Drug Administration website for food manufacturer violations. This federal agency lists food companies that have received warning letters or fines for food safety or labeling violations. If Jason had checked the website, he would have seen that the food manufacturer of the granola bar he ate had numerous sanitation violations and that his risk for an allergic reaction after eating one of its products was very high. While these strategies can minimize the risk for an allergy reaction, it is still not always possible to prevent them. The best strategy Jason used that day was to always have his emergency care kit with him. Luckily his best friend happened to be with him and was able to recognize Jason's symptoms and know how to quickly treat him. But Jason does not wear a MedicAlert bracelet however. Because Jason is now in college, his chance of being with strangers who do not know about his food allergy is very high. If Jason had not been with Steve, he may have not received life-saving treatment before emergency services arrived. Therefore, Jason should wear some type of MedicAlert jewelry so that others can quickly identify the situation and respond appropriately to save his life.

CASE STUDY 2

Melissa is a nine-year-old elementary school student who has a peanut allergy. She was diagnosed when she was two after she ate a peanut butter sandwich, when her lips, tongue, and face became swollen within minutes of eating the sandwich. Melissa's mother brought Melissa to her pediatrician immediately, who administered Benadryl®. Melissa required no further treatment. Melissa's pediatrician subsequently sent her to an allergist, who used skin prick and blood tests to evaluate her for food allergies. Her skin prick tests were positive for both eggs and peanuts, and her blood tests showed an elevated IgE level to peanuts only. The allergist then instructed her mother to put Melissa on an elimination diet, which removed eggs and peanuts from her diet for three weeks, to confirm her diagnosis. After three weeks, Melissa was given a food challenge test with both eggs and peanuts in a hospital to ensure her safety if she experienced a severe reaction. Melissa had swollen lips, tongue, and face immediately after tested with peanuts but had no reaction to eggs. The allergist diagnosed her with a peanut allergy only. Although Melissa has never experienced a severe reaction to eating peanuts, her teachers, cafeteria staff, and classmates have all been made aware that she is allergic to peanuts. School staff were all educated about food allergies and how to treat them. Her school cafeteria also has separate tables for students with food allergies so they may be "safe" from an accidental exposure to their allergen. However, Melissa usually doesn't sit at that table because she has never had a reaction when eating at a regular table before and she likes to sit with her friends. Today Melissa experiences a severe allergic anaphylactic reaction while eating lunch. The teachers recognize her symptoms and immediately administer her EpiPen®, which is kept in the cafeteria. Within minutes she is able to breathe, but emergency services and her parents are called. She is transported to the hospital where she is monitored. It is discovered that she was sitting at a table where a student at the previous lunch period ate a peanut butter sandwich.

Analysis

Allergy reactions can improve or progress to severe as a child ages. In general, most children outgrow a food allergy as they become older. However, this is not the case for most tree nut and peanut allergies, which are rarely outgrown, as Question 14 explores. It remains unclear why a food allergy reaction can progress from mild to severe without any warning or even if it will ever occur. Therefore, anyone with a food allergy should always remember that allergic reactions could progress to severe and take precautions against this possibility. Melissa's school is very proactive about students with food allergies, having a written policy for food allergy management and providing mandatory food allergy training programs to all its staff. In Melissa's case, emergency care was administered quickly and correctly. Teachers and cafeteria staff all recognized Melissa's symptoms of a severe peanut reaction and quickly provided emergency care that undoubtedly saved her life. Studies show that most fatal reactions occur when epinephrine administration is delayed.

But could the reaction have been prevented? It appears that it may have been possible to prevent Melissa's allergy reaction. Two areas of concern in this case involve the appropriate sanitation of tables between lunches and the school's policy of separate lunch tables for those with food allergy. As Question 24 explores, studies show that proper sanitation of tables between lunch periods can remove food allergen residue that may be present on a table, which may then trigger an allergic reaction. The second concern in this case, which involves student choice of where to eat, is an issue that is much more difficult to solve. Melissa knew there was a "safe" table for her to eat at, but she never chose to eat there because she didn't want to be "different" and wanted to be with her friends. As discussed in Question 22, there are pros and cons regarding the separation of students with food allergies from other students for their own safety. Melissa is at an age where peer groups are very important. Melissa didn't want to feel different from everyone else. Individuals with food allergies often feel separated from their classmates because they are different from others, leading to social isolation and potential bullying by others. While Melissa had never experienced a serious food reaction prior to this when exposed to peanuts, the potential for a severe reaction is always possible and she needed to be reminded that a serious reaction could occur at any time. Because of this, she needed encouragement and a reminder about being proactive about her safety. Since Melissa chose to eat at a regular table to be one of the "group," it might be productive for the school to reevaluate its policy of separate allergen-free tables in the cafeteria. One possible solution might be to eliminate allergen-free tables and require strict sanitation procedures of all tables, with systems to ensure this is done before, during, and after all lunch periods. Proper sanitation of tables and other shared objects with soap and water or approved commercial cleaning solutions has proved to be an effective method for removal of potential food allergen residue present on a table or object. Another possible solution might be that all students with food allergies must eat their lunches at allergen-free tables, although this may be very difficult to enforce. Another option could be to allow students with food allergies to eat with their friends at allergen-free tables as long as everyone has an allergen-free lunch. Melissa may also consider presenting a talk about food allergies to her classmates. Educating her classmates may make her feel less "different" and enlist the support of other students to ensure a safe environment for any student with a food allergy.

CASE STUDY 3

Paul is a six-year-old boy who has asthma. He has never been tested for food allergies, but his mother suspects he has an egg allergy because every time he eats eggs he has an asthma attack. His mother brings him to his pediatrician, who sends them to an allergist. The allergist gives Paul a skin prick test, but he tests negative for a food allergy. He is then given blood tests, which also test negative for a food allergy. His mother insists he is allergic to eggs however.

Paul's pediatrician decides that Paul should follow a strict elimination diet, removing the most common food allergens from his diet. Eggs, fish, milk, peanuts, shellfish, tree nuts, soy, and wheat are all eliminated from his diet for three weeks. Because many of the foods that were eliminated from Paul's diet were his favorite foods, his mother saw a registered dietitian. The dietitian evaluated Paul's nutritional needs for his age and planned a well-balanced diet to ensure he continued to grow and not develop any nutritional deficiencies. At the end of three weeks, his mother was instructed to challenge Paul by adding back one food or food group every week to his daily diet. For example, during the first week eggs were added back to his diet. During the second week, he was allowed to have eggs and peanut butter. This diet progression continued until all eliminated foods were added back to his diet. His mother monitored him for the most common signs of a food allergy, which are listed in Question 4.

During the food challenge phase of Paul's diet, his mother discovers that Paul does not have an asthma attack to eggs. However, when he eats wheat, he does experience an asthma attack.

Analysis

As discussed in Question 10, food allergy researchers find a strong link between food allergies and asthma. A 2016 study in the *BIOMED Central Pediatrics Journal* found that young children diagnosed with a food allergy also have an elevated risk for respiratory allergies, such as asthma, during the first five years of life. While studies have been unable to pinpoint the exact number of asthmatics who have food allergies, it is well known that the two often occur together. In Paul's case, his mother had observed that the only time he had an asthma attack was after he ate a meal. This implied that a food was the trigger for his asthma. But food allergy testing did not help to diagnose him. As reviewed in Question

7, food allergy testing is not yet the most accurate way of determining if someone has a food allergy. Skin prick tests with positive results have been identified as being accurate approximately 50–60 percent of the time, meaning a person may not be allergic to the food even though the test shows he or she is. False-negative results are usually considered to be accurate, as they almost always mean there is no allergy. However, as we see in Paul's case, although both Paul's skin prick and blood tests were negative for a food allergy, it is still possible to be allergic.

Paul's mother observed that he had an asthma attack only after eating, indicating a strong connection between what he ate and the asthma attack. Her persistence and recorded food diary of what Paul ate and his symptoms convinced Paul's pediatrician to try a food challenge with him. Typically an oral food challenge is given to confirm a food allergy when other tests are inconclusive. Because Paul was very young and tests results were so inconclusive, his pediatrician felt he would have a difficult time with the oral food challenge test. So he prescribed an elimination diet for three weeks. The food elimination diet is a specific diet that removes all suspected foods for a two- to four-week period of time, which is described in Question 7. If symptoms disappear, it is usually concluded that the eliminated food was the trigger for symptoms. But the allergy or sensitivity is usually confirmed by reintroducing eliminated foods one at a time into the diet and monitoring for a return of symptoms. In Paul's case, his pediatrician decided to remove the most common food allergens from his diet, as explored in Question 1. As we saw, this continued persistence for testing Paul was appropriate. After Paul underwent the reintroduction phase of eliminated foods, it was discovered that Paul did have a food allergy. However, it was not to the food his mother thought it was, highlighting the fact that many times family members or individuals can identify the wrong food for their symptoms. The discovery of Paul's actual food allergy also stresses the importance of undergoing a thorough evaluation for food allergies by a medical professional. In Paul's case, his mother always gave him eggs with toast or another wheat product. The elimination diet quickly identified the specific food he was really allergic to. Elimination diets and food challenges continue to be the most accurate testing methods available to date for confirming a food allergy.

CASE STUDY 4

Mary is a very healthy 70-year-old woman, who loves milk and has always included milk, cheese, and yogurt in her daily diet. She has been healthy all her life and never had any allergies to her food or environment. She does not have any problems with her gastrointestinal system and eats everything she likes. But Mary began to notice that, when she turned 60, her abdomen would become bloated, and she would have flatulence whenever she ate or drank any food made from milk. She also began to experience diarrhea if she ate or drank more than one glass of milk or one cup of yogurt a day. Mary decided to eliminate all dairy foods from her diet and now finds her bloating and gas have gone away as long as she maintains a dairy-free diet.

At her annual checkup, Mary mentioned her symptoms to her primary care physician, who scheduled a lactose intolerance blood test for her. Mary's test results showed that she was indeed lactose intolerant. Mary has continued to eliminate all dairy from her diet and no longer experiences any symptoms.

Analysis

It is very common for individuals to become lactose intolerant as they age. Recall from Questions 2, 5, and 11 that food intolerances almost always involve the gastrointestinal tract and are the result of inadequate digestion. They are not allergic reactions, however, and rarely life threatening. But food intolerances can have serious health implications if left untreated. In general, a food intolerance is usually caused by the absence or deficiency of a digestive enzyme in the gastrointestinal tract. Digestive enzymes are responsible for breaking down foods into usable components the body needs for health. When enzyme production decreases or is absent in the digestive tract, food remains undigested in the gastrointestinal tract, where it then undergoes a partially digested process of bacterial fermentation instead. This fermentation process produces the gases hydrogen sulfide, nitric oxide, ammonia, and methane. These gases then produce symptoms of abdominal pain, bloating, constipation, diarrhea, or flatulence.

Mary appears to be lactose intolerant, which is one of the most common food intolerances worldwide, as seen in Question 16. An estimated 30–50 million Americans are lactose intolerant. Question 11 also highlighted the fact that lactose intolerance tends to become more common as individuals age because the production of the lactase enzyme, which is necessary to digest the milk sugar lactose found in milk and dairy-based foods, decreases with age. Decreased enzyme production can occur because of age, chronic health conditions, a viral illness, or genetic factors. There are three types of lactose intolerances: primary, secondary, and congenital. Primary lactose intolerance is diagnosed when someone has a decreased amount of lactose available in his or her gastrointestinal system, usually as a result of the aging process. Secondary lactose intolerance occurs after a viral illness, which can temporarily decrease the production of lactase until the gastrointestinal system heals. Often individuals with secondary lactose intolerance are able to eat milk and milk-based foods without symptoms once their gastrointestinal tract heals. Congenital lactose intolerance occurs because of a genetic defect that prevents the digestion of the sugar galactose, which is part of the lactose sugar molecule found in milk.

Mary most likely has a primary lactose intolerance because her symptoms after drinking or eating milk and milk-based foods occurred only as she became older. She also reported that she improved and had not symptoms as long as she avoided milk and milk-based foods. Like food allergies and the majority of food sensitivities, diagnostic testing for lactose intolerance is reliable about 60 percent of the time. As discussed in Question 8, lactose intolerance is usually diagnosed in older adults using the hydrogen breath test or lactose tolerance blood test. The hydrogen blood test measures the amount of hydrogen found in the breath over a specified period of time after drinking a lactose solution. The lactose tolerance blood test measures the amount of glucose in the blood two hours after drinking a lactose solution. Elimination diets may also be used to determine if milk is causing symptoms. In Mary's case, she already learned that milk and milk-based foods caused her symptoms and that eliminating these foods prevented them. But she did decide to confirm her self-made diagnosis by having a lactose blood intolerance test. While she feels she eats very healthy, it may be beneficial for her to discuss her diet with a registered dietitian to replace the nutrients she loses from milk and milk-based foods in her daily diet. As reviewed in Question 23, elimination of a food group can lead to nutrient deficiencies. Eliminating milk may lead to deficiencies of calcium, pantothenic acid, phosphorus, and riboflavin as well as vitamins A, D, and B_{12}.

CASE STUDY 5

Anthony is a 59-year-old male, who is very healthy and has a good appetite. In the past, he always ate everything he wanted and did not have any seasonal allergies.

About five years ago Anthony caught a virus that was making the rounds at his workplace. His symptoms included a slight fever, weakness, nausea, diarrhea, and "stomach pains." He was very sick for three days, and it took him about two weeks to recover enough to feel normal and get back to eating his usual foods. But he now reports he has a "sensitive" stomach and is alternating between symptoms of diarrhea and constipation. He also notices he feels extreme joint pain after he eats corn or any foods that contain corn.

Anthony visited his primary care doctor, who did routine blood work. This included complete blood chemistry and complete blood count panels to assess if he had anemia or any other serious health issues. His lab results were all normal, and his physician felt no further testing was necessary. His doctor recommended he avoid corn and take Miralax, an osmotic laxative, when he constipated, and Imodium, an antidiarrheal medicine, when he experienced diarrhea.

Anthony does not want to be on these medications and feels there is another reason for his symptoms because he never had a problem with his gastrointestinal tract before the virus. He decides to see a registered dietitian, who can test him for food sensitivities to determine what is causing his symptoms.

Analysis

This case highlights how food sensitivities can begin and progress into chronic health conditions. As Question 12 explores, the gastrointestinal system has more of an impact on the immune system and overall health of humans than ever realized before. We now know that an estimated 70 percent of the entire immune system resides in the intestine. Viruses can disrupt the integrity and function of the gastrointestinal tract. This in turn can lead to a condition known as dysbiosis, also called "leaky gut," which causes damage to the intestinal junctions of the gastrointestinal cells. The "loosening" of gastrointestinal junctions, also called "holes," allows undigested foods and toxins to enter into the bloodstream. Normally tight gastrointestinal cell junctions would prevent this from happening. Viruses can also cause an imbalance of good bacteria and bad bacteria in the intestines, which can be worsened if antibiotics are taken. Bacterial imbalances affect the functioning of the gastrointestinal tract, which can cause symptoms. Typical symptoms, outlined in Question 6, include Anthony's symptoms of constipation and diarrhea. This case also highlights how difficult it can be to receive a correct diagnosis. Many people who suffer with chronic sensitivities often have "normal" test results when seen by their primary care doctors or specialists. This can be extremely frustrating for patients, who often develop a chronic condition and sometimes become sicker. As discussed in Question 12, there are many different causes for food sensitivities, and they remain very difficult to diagnose.

In Anthony's case, it appears the virus he had damaged his gastrointestinal cells. It would seem that the junctions between his gastrointestinal cells were "loosened up," allowing substances to pass through into the bloodstream that ordinarily would not be allowed to do so. It is highly likely that "partially" digested food substances were passing through these gastrointestinal "holes" and then carried by the blood throughout the body. It is possible these particles were deposited in his joints, giving Anthony extreme joint pain because they did not belong there. His joint pain could also be caused by an overall systemic inflammation, which can occur when substances circulating throughout the body should not be there. However, it doesn't explain why only corn gives him pain when he does not notice this from other foods and why he has alternating symptoms of constipation and diarrhea. The registered dietitian Anthony visits is trained and skilled in assessing and counseling patients with food sensitivities. After an initial nutrition assessment, his dietitian recommends IgE and mediator release blood (MRT) testing along with the LEAP (Lifestyle, Eating, and Performance) diet. As we saw in Questions 7 and 9, more than one testing method is often used to diagnose any type of adverse food reaction because of the unreliability of current testing methods. Immunoglobulin E antibodies are measured because elevated IgE levels indicate an allergic reaction. IgE food tests measure the amount of IgE antibodies produced by the blood of a patient to specific foods. MRT blood tests evaluate different foods and additives and measures the release of cytokines, histamine, leukotrienes, and prostaglandins, which are mast cell mediators released by white blood cells in response to inflammation and allergic reactions, in a patient's blood. Elevations of these inflammatory biomarkers indicate an allergic response to that specific food or additive. The LEAP diet is then used to confirm the accuracy of the MRT test results. For instance, MRT results are categorized into highly reactive, moderately reactive, and low-reactive foods. These foods are then eliminated from the diet for a period of time and then challenged one by one until a complete pattern of sensitivity is identified.

Anthony's IgE levels were normal and did not indicate he had a food allergy. However, his MRT results showed he was sensitive to corn, milk, and strawberries. Anthony's dietitian planned his LEAP diet carefully so he would follow it and not be too bored by the lack of food variety. Anthony carefully followed the diet and learned that he was sensitive to milk and corn but had no symptoms if he ate strawberries. He also found he had joint pain when he ate chic peas. This finding highlights the possibility that a food that is not suspected or low reactive on the MRT test can still be discovered to provoke symptoms, which is why MRT tests and the LEAP diet are often combined to ensure accuracy. Anthony eliminated milk, chic peas, and corn from his diet and noticed that the pain in his joints stopped. But he continued to have alternating symptoms of constipation and diarrhea.

Anthony's dietitian then recommended a vitamin D blood test and specialized microbiome testing to assess the integrity and exact bacterial balance of his gastrointestinal system. Low vitamin D levels are known to increase intestinal permeability, which in turn may cause a "leaky" gut. There are many different companies that perform microbiome testing, which involves collecting a stool sample from the patient that is then tested for bacterial composition. His test results showed low vitamin D levels and a bacterial imbalance. His dietitian prescribed a vitamin D supplement daily and a specific probiotic supplement that supported the restoration of his intestinal bacteria to healthy levels. The dietitian also recommended a glutathione supplement to restore and heal the gastrointestinal junctions in his gastrointestinal tract that were damaged by the virus. After four weeks, Anthony's symptoms of constipation and diarrhea resolved. Anthony's maintenance diet plan recommended that Anthony increase his vegetable consumption to at least four servings per day and fruit servings to no more than three. The plan also recommended organic and non-GMO foods, as conventional crops and GMO foods have been linked in some studies to increased risk for intestinal permeability or leaky gut, as discussed in Question 12. Finally, Anthony's diet plan advised that foods with a high sugar content be eliminated because sugar promotes bacterial imbalance in the gastrointestinal tract. Many patients who develop symptoms after a virus are often able to eat foods that caused their symptoms after their intestinal tract fully heals. One year later, Anthony is symptom free and able to eat corn and chic peas again. He remains sensitive to milk however.

Glossary

Adjuvant: substance used in vaccines to make them more potent and increase an immune reaction.

Allergic eosinophilic gastroenteritis: overabundance of eosinophils in the lining of the digestive tract.

Anaphylaxis: immune response affecting the respiratory system, causing difficulty breathing or swelling of the throat and often fatal.

Antibody: protein produced in the blood and used by the immune system to fight foreign substances and protect the body.

Antigen: foreign substance that induces an immune response by the body, usually producing antibodies.

Antigen leukocyte cellular antibody test (ALCAT): test used to identify food sensitivities.

Basophil: white blood cell.

Bradykinins: inflammatory mediator.

Cross contamination: when a small amount of a food allergen accidentally gets onto another food that does not have allergens.

Cytokine: inflammatory mediator.

Dysbiosis: imbalance of gastrointestinal bacteria.

Elimination diet: specific diet plan that removes all suspected foods for a two- to four-week period to help in the diagnosis of food sensitivities.

Enzymes: protein molecules that induce and control the rate of specific chemical reactions in the body.

Eosinophil: white blood cell.

Epinephrine: also called adrenaline, a hormone secreted by the adrenal gland in response to stress that increases heart rate and blood pressure while relaxing lung bronchi to ease breathing difficulties.

EpiPen®: epinephrine medication in an auto-injector device that administers the correct dose of epinephrine to an individual during an allergic reaction.

FALCPA: Food Allergen Labeling and Consumer Protection Act.

Food allergy: when the immune system mistakenly identifies a specific food as a threat and overreacts by attacking a protein component found in the food.

Food-dependent, exercise-induced anaphylaxis: a rare food sensitivity that occurs only if an individual exercises within a one- to four-hour period before or after eating a specific food he or she is sensitive to.

Food intolerance: adverse reaction to a food that does not involve the immune system, is not usually life threatening, and tends to involve the digestive tract.

Food protein–induced enterocolitis syndrome: a non-IgE-mediated food reaction that affects the gastrointestinal system and does not involve an immune system release of antibodies.

Food protein–induced proctocolitis: also known as allergic or eosinophilic proctocolitis or protein intolerance, typically occurring within the first few months of a susceptible infant's life; considered an allergy, rather than a sensitivity, because of an abnormal response to a food protein.

Food sensitivity: negative reactions to a food or food component, such as food additive; sometimes involves the immune system but may also affect the brain, gastrointestinal system, joints, skin, and respiratory tract.

Fructan: short-chain carbohydrate found primarily in fruits, vegetables, and grain.

Fructose malabsorption: when fructose cannot be absorbed and accumulates in the intestine.

Galactosemia: genetic disorder that affects the ability to process the simple sugar galactose, which is part of the larger lactose sugar molecule that is found in milk and dairy foods.

GALT system: gut-associated lymphoid tissue in the intestine that decreases the permeability of the intestine and is a backup immune defense system.

Gluten: substance found in wheat.

Gluten-sensitive enteropathy: also called celiac sprue, it is classified as a gluten intolerance or wheat allergy.

GMO: genetically modified organism.

GMPs: good manufacturing practices.

GRAS: generally recognized as safe food ingredients approved by the U.S. Food and Drug Administration as safe for human consumption.

Hapten: a molecule that elicits an immune response.

Hereditary fructose intolerance (HFI): deficiency of the enzyme aldolase B, which is produced by the liver.

Histamine: inflammatory mediator.

Hydrogen breath test: measures hydrogen present in the breath and used to diagnose fructose, lactose, sucrose, and sorbitol intolerances, and SIBO.

IgG, IgA, IgE, IgM, IgD: Five immunoglobulin antibodies produced by the human immune system. IgG and IgM are the primary antibodies produced to attack bacterial, pathogen, and viral infections. IgA antibodies also attack bacteria, pathogens, and viruses but only in the gastrointestinal tract and breathing passages. IgE and IgD antibodies are specialty antibodies that are rarely produced. IgE antibodies are produced to fight parasite infections and increase during food allergy reactions. IgD antibody function remains unknown at this time.

Immunoglobulin: proteins in the blood and cells of the immune system.

Lactose tolerance blood test: blood test used to diagnose lactose intolerance.

Leaky gut: also called increased intestinal permeability, gastrointestinal cells that become loose and create "holes" through which toxins, undigested foods, and bacteria can pass.

LEAP diet: Lifestyle, eating, and performance diet tailored specifically to the individual to evaluate food sensitivities.

Leukocyte: white blood cells.

Leukotriene: inflammatory mediator.

Lymphocyte response assay: test used to identify food sensitivities.

Lymphocytes: white blood cells, classified as T cells and B cells. B cells form in the bone marrow and consist of mast cells and basophils. T cells assist B cells by sending out signals to eosinophils to fight infections.

Mast cells: cell filled with basophils that release chemicals during allergic reactions.

Mediator release blood test (MRT): test used to diagnose food sensitivities.

NSAIDS: nonsteroidal anti-inflammatory drugs.

Oral allergy syndrome: allergic reaction to a protein found in environmental pollens.

Oral food challenge: used when other allergy testing is unclear in the presence of symptoms. Suspected allergenic foods are ingested under strict medical supervision and reactions monitored. Three kinds of oral food challenges are used: double-blind, placebo-controlled food challenge, single-blind food challenge, and open blind food challenge.

Phagocyte: white blood cell.

Prostaglandin: inflammatory mediator.

RAST: radioallergosorbent test that uses a radioactive substance to identify IgE in the blood, signifying an allergic reaction.

Serum sickness: an allergic reaction to serum antitoxins found in vaccine ingredients.

Skin prick test: also called scratch testing, an allergy testing method that uses a drop of solution containing different common food allergens that is placed onto the skin of the patient. A small plastic needle is used to gently scratch the skin, allowing a small amount of the solution to enter the skin just below the surface. If a raised white bump surrounded by a small circle of itchy red skin occurs within 30 minutes, the test indicates a positive reaction and an allergy to that particular food. If there is no skin reaction, the test is considered negative.

Small intestinal bacterial overgrowth: also called SIBO, an abnormal amount of bacteria in the small intestine that is normally found in the colon.

Sulfite-induced asthma: adverse reaction to sulfites found in foods or medications.

Type I hypersensitivity: associated with severe reactions and food allergies.

Type II hypersensitivity: usually IgG mediated but has not been associated with food reactions.

Type III hypersensitivity: affects either the body in general or specific individual organs. Reactions may be delayed after antigen exposure.

Type IV hypersensitivity: thought to be possible root cause for many autoimmune diseases. Symptoms usually occur 48–72 hours after antigen exposure, and this delayed reaction is thought to be tied to food sensitivities because of the length of time it takes for symptoms to appear.

Directory of Resources

BOOKS AND ARTICLES

Behrhorst, Dana. 2014. "The Pros and Cons to Banning Allergens from Schools." August 25, 2014. PeanutAllergy.com. https://www.peanutallergy.com/articles/the-pros-and-cons-to-banning-allergens-from-schools.

Bergmann, K. C., and Ring, J. (eds). 2014. "History of Allergy." *Chemical Immunology and Allergy*. 100: 109–119.

Buchanan, B. 2001. "Genetic Engineering and the Allergy Issue." *Plant Physiology*. 126: 1, 5–7.

D'Brant, J. n.d. "The Shikmate Pathway, the Microbiome, and Disease: Health Effects of GMOS on Humans." http://teca.fao.org/sites/default/files/comments/files/GMO%2CShikimate_pathway_gut_flora_and_health.pdf.

Fischer, R., McGhee, J. R., Lan Vu, H., Atkinson, T. P., Jackson, R. J., Tome, D., et al. 2005. "Oral and Nasal Sensitization Promote Distinct Immune Responses and Lung Reactivity in a Mouse Model of Peanut Allergy." *American Journal of Pathology*. 167: 6, 1621–1630.

Fraser, Heather. 2011. *The Peanut Allergy Epidemic: What's Causing It and How to Stop It*. Second Edition. New York, NY: Skyhorse Publishing.

Gavura, S. 2012. "IgG Food Intolerance Tests: What Does the Science Say?" February 2, 2102. Science Based Medicine. https://sciencebasedmedicine.org/igg-food-intolerance-tests-what-does-the-science-say/.

Hong, X., Hao, K., Ladd-Acosta, C., Hansen, K. D., Tsai, H. J., Liu, X., et al. 2015. "Genome-Wide Association Study Identifies Peanut Allergy-Specific Loci and Evidence of Epigenetic Mediation in US Children." *Nat Commun.* 6: 6304, 1–12. doi:10.1038/ncomms7304.

Jackson, Mark. 2006. *Allergy: The History of a Modern Malady*. London, UK: Reaktion Books.

Jacobson, M. 2006. *Allergy: The History of a Modern Malady*. London, UK: Reaktion Books.

Martin, L. J., Hua, H., Collins, M. H., Abonia, J. P., Biagini Myers, J. M., Eby, M., et al. 2018. "Eosinophilic Esophagitis (EoE) Genetic Susceptibility Is Mediated by Synergistic Interactions between EoE-Specific and General Atopic Disease Loci." *Journal of Allergy and Clinical Immunology*. 141: 5, 1690–1698.

More, D. 2018. "Boiled Peanuts May Be the Key to Curing Peanut Allergies." June 20, 2018. Very Well Health. https://www.verywellhealth.com/boiled-peanuts-may-cure-allergy-83175.

Muraro, A., and Roberts, G. (eds). 2014. "European Academy of Allergy and Clinical Immunology. Food Allergy and Anaphylaxis Guidelines, Supplementary Materials." https://www.eaaci.org/attachments/Food%20Allergy%20Supplementary%20V1.pdf.

Prescott, S. L., Pawankar, R., Allen, K. J., Campbell, D. E., Sinn, J.K.H., Fiocchi, A. et al., 2013. "A Global Survey of Changing Patterns of Good Allergy Burden in Children." *The World Health Organization Journal*. 6: 1, 21.

Profet, M. 1991. "The Function of Allergy: Immunological Defense against Toxins." *The Quarterly Review of Biology*. 66: 1, 23–62.

Ramanathan, M., and Mims, J. 2017. "Allergy for the Otolaryngologist." *Otolaryngologic Clinics of North America, Clinics Review Articles*. 50: 6, xvii-xviii.

Richet, C. R. Nobel Lecture, December 11, 1913. NobelPrize.org. Nobel Media AB 2018. https://www.nobelprize.org/prizes/medicine/1913/richet/lecture/

Royal College of Physicians. 2003. *Allergy: The Unmet need: A Blueprint for Better Patient Care*.

Sicherer, Scott H. 2013. *Food Allergies: A Complete Guide for Eating When Your Life Depends on It*. Baltimore, MD: Johns Hopkins University Press.

Sicherer, S.H., Muñoz-Furlong, A., Godbold, J. H., and Sampson, H. A.. 2010. "US Prevalence of Self Reported Peanut, Tree Nut, and Sesame Allergy; 11 Year Follow Up." *Journal of Allergy and Clinical Immunology*. 125: 6, 1322–1326.

Wighton, Kate. 2016. "Feeding Babies Egg and Peanut May Prevent Food Allergy." September 20, 2016. Imperial College London, Imperial Today. https://www.imperial.ac.uk/news/174630/feeding-babies-peanut-prevent-food-allergy/.

Wong, G. 2011. "Patterns of Food Allergy outside Europe." *Clinical and Translational Allergy*. Suppl. 1: S6.

Zopf, Y., Eckhart, G. H., Raithel, M., Baenkler, H. W., and Silbermann, A.. 2009. "The Differential Diagnosis of Food Intolerance." *Deutsches Arzteblatt International*. 106: 21, 359–370.

ORGANIZATIONS

American Academy of Allergy Asthma & Immunology
http://www.aaaai.org/

American Partnership for Eosinophilic Disorders
http://apfed.org

Asthma and Allergy Foundation of America
http://asthmaandallergies.org

Beyond Celiac
https://www.beyondceliac.org

Food Allergy & Anaphylaxis Connection Team
http://www.foodallergyawareness.org

Food Allergy Research & Education
https://www.foodallergy.org

Gluten Intolerance Group
https://www.gluten.org

National Center for Biotechnology Information
https://www.ncbi.nlm.nih.gov

U.S. Food & Drug Administration
https://www.fda.gov/

World Allergy Organization
http://www.worldallergy.org

WEBSITES

Anaphylaxis Campaign
https://www.anaphylaxis.org.uk

EpiPen
https://www.epipen.com/-/media/files/epipen/howtouseepipenautoinjector.pdf

Food Allergy Research and Resource Program. University of Nebraska-Lincoln, Institute of Agriculture and Natural Resources
https://farrp.unl.edu

Food Reactions
https://foodreactions.org

Harvard Health Publishing, Harvard Medical School
https://www.health.harvard.edu

Hello Peanut
https://www.hello-peanut.com

Kids with Food Allergies
https://community.kidswithfoodallergies.org

MedicAlert Foundation
https://www.medicalert.org

Soil and Health Library
https://www.soilandhealth.org/wp-content/uploads/02/0201hyglibcat/020108.coca.pdf

U.S. National Library of Medicine, National Institutes of Health
https://www.ncbi.nlm.nih.gov

Index

About the Author

Alice C. Richer, RDN, MBA, LDN, is a registered and licensed dietitian, advanced certified functional nutritionist, and certified medical writer who has been helping patients improve their nutrition habits and overall wellness for over 25 years. Alice received her Bachelor of Science from the University of Rhode Island and Master of Business Administration from Boston College, completed her dietetic internship at the Beth Israel Hospital in Boston, and completed certifications from the American Medical Writers Association and Next Level Functional Nutrition. She is currently studying nutrigenomics. She is the author of *Student Guide to Health: Nutrition and Physical Fitness* (Vol. 2), *Food Allergies*, and coauthor of *Understanding the Antioxidant Controversy*. She practices at Spaulding Outpatient Centers in Massachusetts and is the team nutritionist for the New England Revolution soccer team.